# IAMSE Manuals

**Editor-in-Chief**
Steven M. Crooks, Western Michigan University Homer Stryker
Kalamazoo, MI, USA

**Editorial Board**

Jongpil Cheon, Texas Tech University
Lubbock, TX, USA

Peter G. M. de Jong, Leiden University Medical Center
Leiden, The Netherlands

David W. Mullins, Dartmouth Geisel School of Medicine
Hanover, NH, USA

Thom F. Oostendorp, Radboud University Medical Center
Nijmegen, The Netherlands

The book series IAMSE Manuals is established to rapidly deploy the latest developments and best evidence-based examples in medical education, offering all who teach in healthcare the most current information to succeed in their task by publishing short "how-to-guides" on a variety of topics relevant to medical teaching. The series aims to make the best and latest evidence-based methods for teaching in medical education to educators around the world, to improve the quality of teaching in healthcare education, and to establish greater interest in the teaching of the medical sciences.

More information about this series at http://www.springer.com/series/16034

Ivo de Boer • Femmie de Vegt • Helma Pluk
Mieke Latijnhouwers

# Rubrics – a tool for feedback and assessment viewed from different perspectives

Enhancing learning and assessment quality

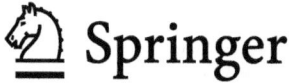

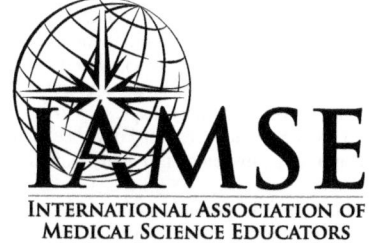

Ivo de Boer
Center for Innovation in Medical Education
Leiden University Medical Center
Leiden, The Netherlands

Helma Pluk
Department of Biochemistry
Radboudumc Health Academy
Radboud University Medical Centre
Nijmegen, The Netherlands

Femmie de Vegt
Department for Health Evidence
Radboud University Medical Centre
Nijmegen, The Netherlands

Mieke Latijnhouwers
Education Support Center
Wageningen University
Wageningen, The Netherlands

ISSN 2673-9291         ISSN 2673-9305   (electronic)
IAMSE Manuals
ISBN 978-3-030-86847-5        ISBN 978-3-030-86848-2   (eBook)
https://doi.org/10.1007/978-3-030-86848-2

© The Author(s), under exclusive license to Springer Nature Switzerland AG 2021
This work is subject to copyright. All rights are solely and exclusively licensed by the Publisher, whether the whole or part of the material is concerned, specifically the rights of translation, reprinting, reuse of illustrations, recitation, broadcasting, reproduction on microfilms or in any other physical way, and transmission or information storage and retrieval, electronic adaptation, computer software, or by similar or dissimilar methodology now known or hereafter developed.
The use of general descriptive names, registered names, trademarks, service marks, etc. in this publication does not imply, even in the absence of a specific statement, that such names are exempt from the relevant protective laws and regulations and therefore free for general use.
The publisher, the authors and the editors are safe to assume that the advice and information in this book are believed to be true and accurate at the date of publication. Neither the publisher nor the authors or the editors give a warranty, expressed or implied, with respect to the material contained herein or for any errors or omissions that may have been made. The publisher remains neutral with regard to jurisdictional claims in published maps and institutional affiliations.

This Springer imprint is published by the registered company Springer Nature Switzerland AG
The registered company address is: Gewerbestrasse 11, 6330 Cham, Switzerland

# Preface

In this how-to guide for rubrics, we describe how to use rubrics for assessment and feedback. The manual is addressed to teachers, students and educational advisors in higher education such as universities and higher colleges.

In Chap. 1 we start with a definition and description of rubrics and how to design and implement a rubric for your own education. In Chap. 2 we describe four best practices in using rubrics for a written assignment, for an oral presentation, for collaboration skills and for clinical skills. The focus is on the feedback purposes and grading of assignments with rubrics. Examples from several Dutch universities are discussed.

In Chap. 3 we portray perspectives on rubrics from different stakeholders that are involved in higher education: students, teachers, educational advisors and curriculum managers.

In this manual we hope to sketch the demands that need to be met in order to successfully create a culture where rubrics are used as a tool to enhance feedback to students and improve the quality of grading of diverse assignments. We hope it will inspire you!

| | |
|---|---:|
| Leiden, The Netherlands | Ivo de Boer |
| Nijmegen, The Netherlands | Femmie de Vegt |
| Nijmegen, The Netherlands | Helma Pluk |
| Wageningen, The Netherlands | Mieke Latijnhouwers |

# Acknowledgements

We are grateful to all students, teachers and educational advisors we have worked with in the last years in developing and using rubrics for assessment and feedback. Your comments, advice and experiences have been very important to enhance the use of rubrics in our educational settings and inspired many of the practical tips in this manual. We would like to thank Dr. N.A. Gruis (LUMC), Dr. W.T. Steegenga (WU), S. Zijlstra, MSc MA (WU), Dr. J. Gulikers (WU), Dr. M. Coppens (WU), Dr I. Palm (WU), E. Rasenberg, MSc (RU), and L. Rietveld, MSc (RU), for their rubrics, their experience and advice. Finally we would like to thank Dr. Thom Oostendorp (RU), for his critical view on this manual and his advice for improvement.

# Contents

**1 Rubrics: A Start** .................................................... 1
    1.1 What Is a Rubric? ............................................. 2
        1.1.1 Format ................................................. 2
        1.1.2 Purpose and Applications ............................ 3
    1.2 Checklist for Designing a Rubric .............................. 7
        1.2.1 Types of Rubric ....................................... 7
        1.2.2 Criteria ............................................... 7
        1.2.3 Rating Scale .......................................... 8
        1.2.4 Performance Descriptors ............................ 8
        1.2.5 Feedback .............................................. 9
        1.2.6 Marking, Scores, Norms and Grades ................. 11
    1.3 How to Use a Rubric? ......................................... 12
        1.3.1 The Assessment Process: Choices to Be Made ...... 12
        1.3.2 Evaluation and Improvement ......................... 14
    References ...................................................... 15

**2 Rubrics: Best Practices** ........................................... 17
    2.1 Rubric for a Written Assignment .............................. 18
        2.1.1 Context in Which the Rubric Is Developed and Used ...... 18
        2.1.2 Construction of the Rubric for a Written Assignment ..... 19
        2.1.3 Use of the Rubric in Practice ........................ 21
    2.2 Rubric for an Oral Presentation ............................... 22
        2.2.1 Context in Which the Rubric Is Developed and Used ...... 23
        2.2.2 Construction of the Rubric for an Oral Presentation ...... 23
        2.2.3 Use of the Rubric in Practice ........................ 25
    2.3 Rubric for Collaboration Skills ............................... 29
        2.3.1 Context in Which the Rubric Is Developed and Used ...... 29
        2.3.2 Construction of the Rubric for Collaboration Skills ...... 30
        2.3.3 Use of the Rubric in Practice ........................ 30
    2.4 Rubric for Clinical Skills ..................................... 31
        2.4.1 Context in Which the Rubric Is Developed and Used ...... 35

|   |   | 2.4.2 Construction of the Rubric to Assess Clinical Skills | 35 |
|---|---|---|---|
|   |   | 2.4.3 Use of the Rubrics in Practice | 39 |
|   | References | | 40 |
| 3 | **Perspectives on Rubrics** | | 41 |
|   | 3.1 | Perspectives of Students | 41 |
|   | 3.2 | Perspectives of Educational Advisors | 43 |
|   | 3.3 | Perspectives of Teachers | 44 |
|   | 3.4 | Perspectives of Curriculum Coordinators and Managers | 46 |
|   | References | | 48 |

**Conclusion** . . . . . . . . . . . . . . . . . . . . . . . . . . . . . . . . . . . . . . . . . . . . . . . . 49

# Chapter 1
# Rubrics: A Start

## Contents

1.1 What Is a Rubric?................................................................. 2
    1.1.1 Format...................................................................... 2
    1.1.2 Purpose and Applications............................................ 3
1.2 Checklist for Designing a Rubric........................................... 7
    1.2.1 Types of Rubric........................................................... 7
    1.2.2 Criteria....................................................................... 7
    1.2.3 Rating Scale................................................................ 8
    1.2.4 Performance Descriptors............................................. 8
    1.2.5 Feedback.................................................................... 9
    1.2.6 Marking, Scores, Norms and Grades........................... 10
1.3 How to Use a Rubric?.......................................................... 12
    1.3.1 The Assessment Process: Choices to Be Made............. 12
    1.3.2 Evaluation and Improvement...................................... 14
References................................................................................ 15

**Abstract** A rubric is an instrument for guidance and/or assessment that has the shape of a table with evaluation criteria to the left and a scale with different levels of achievement on top, plus descriptors in each cell. With these descriptors each criterion and level (of performance) is made explicit.

    A rubric helps students understand what they are expected to learn and delivers and facilitates self-assessment and peer evaluation. To assessors, rubrics provide guidance on how to evaluate and mark, and offer an efficient means of providing pre-coded feedback.

    Developing a rubric is a team effort, discussing what you value in performance and how this relates to the intended learning outcomes. It usually takes some iterations of using, evaluating and improving before a rubric fully fits the needs of assessors and students. This chapter provides you with practical advice and guides you through several considerations to take into account.

## 1.1 What Is a Rubric?

For evaluation of student performance, both formative feedback and summative assessment are essential parts in educational/assessment programs. Their purpose is threefold:

1. Inform students where they stand with respect to the learning outcomes they need to master,
2. Inform teachers what might need extra attention in their teaching and supervision and
3. Underpin decisions on study progress and graduation of students.

Besides written exams where students answer questions with open or closed response formats, evaluation of all kinds of products and behaviour is a significant component in many assessment programs. To evaluate these, a rubric is a helpful instrument (Stevens & Levi, 2013; Reddy & Andrade, 2010). In short, a rubric is a specific type of assessment instrument that instructs how to value performance as seen in a product or observed behaviour. The next paragraphs explain what a rubric looks like and how to use it.

### 1.1.1 Format

A rubric typically has the form of a table, with a scale representing different **levels of achievement** across the top row and **evaluation criteria** down the first column (Fig. 1.1). Each cell in the table contains a short **description** of the characteristics

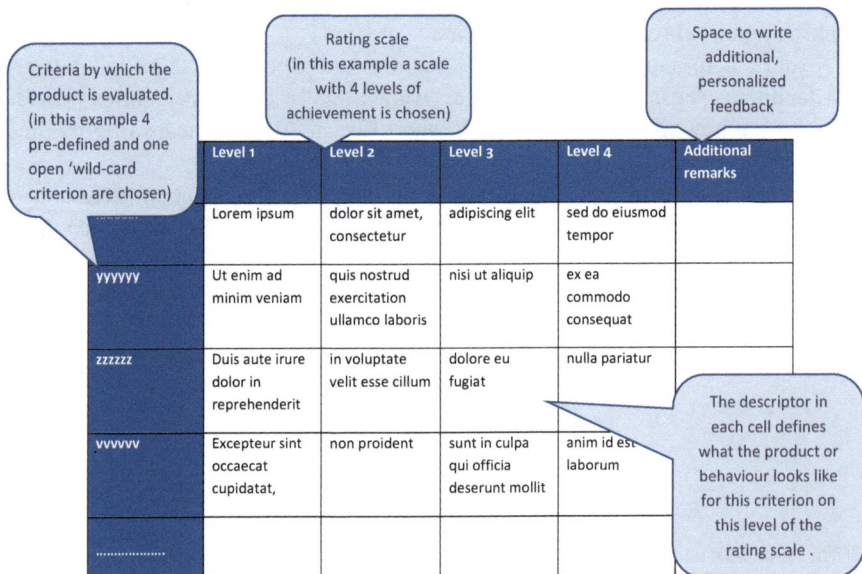

**Fig. 1.1** A rubric typically has the form of a table that combines criteria (rows) with a rating scale (columns) and descriptions of performance (cells)

of a product or behaviour associated with a specific evaluation criterion and achievement level. In this way, a rubric makes explicit how that product or behaviour is valued. If the rubric is used for scoring, scores can be attributed to the descriptions in the table. This score can vary for different criteria, or can be fixed per column of the rating scale shown on top of the table.

In addition to the pre-defined content, rubrics often have space for free-text remarks from the assessor—either as an extra '*wild-card*' criterion or as a comments field for each of the pre-defined criteria. These can be used for supplementary personalized feedback and can contribute to the scoring as well.

There are two main types of rubrics: analytical and holistic. Analytical rubrics discern multiple achievement levels for each criterion, whereas holistic rubrics contain one level per criterion (see also Sect. 1.2.1). Figure 1.1 shows the general characteristic format of a rubric. Figure 1.2 shows an example of an analytical rubric used for a writing assignment. Figure 1.3 depicts a holistic rubric used for a writing component in an internship. Note that there is no standard format; variations are possible on several levels.

## 1.1.2 Purpose and Applications

Rubrics serve different purposes for the different stakeholders involved in the assessment. See Table 1.1. Overall, the descriptors in a rubric provide language to talk about the task to all involved. This affects several aspects of the learning, teaching and assessment process. A rubric helps students understand what they are expected to learn; it serves a feed-up function (Hattie & Timperley, 2007) for the assignment. In view of the concept of '*assessment for learning*' (Martinez & Lipson, 1989), the most important purpose of rubrics is that it is a means to provide students with more **formative feedback** in an efficient way. By indicating which descriptors in each cell of the rubric apply to the students' performance, it informs them how their product or performance is valued. And by looking at the rubric, students can also see for themselves what they could do to further improve. Furthermore, a rubric can facilitate **self-assessment** and **peer evaluation**. In this way rubrics help students to gain insight in their level of development and to direct their further learning (feed-forward function) (Hattie & Timperley, 2007). Learning to evaluate and steer learning are key when students develop into professionals that need to be able to apply self-directed learning (Garrison, 1997) and to keep developing and remain competent during their professional career.

For teachers (or other assessors) rubrics provide **guidance on how to evaluate and mark**. This is especially valuable for unexperienced assessors or when assessing with a team. Designing a rubric together requires dialogue and coordination amongst all assessors involved. Teachers need to make explicit what they value as important, what they define as adequate or insufficient, and what they expect students to achieve. So, a rubric will help you to make the assessment more **transparent** and could also inform what to pay attention to in teaching. Furthermore it can improve **validity** of the assessment: it is much easier to check whether the way you evaluate matches the learning outcomes and teaching activities if you make explicit

*Courtesy of Dr. Giel Bosman and Dr. Thom Oostendorp, Radboud University Medical Center in Nijmegen, The Netherlands*

| | Insufficient; needs rewriting | Deficient; can be compensated | Sufficient / Good | Exemplary |
|---|---|---|---|---|
| Title | Absent or does not match content | Gives impression of content 1pt | Provides information on background and content 2pt | Is appealing and provides information on background, content and main conclusions 3pt |
| Introduction | Does not provide background knowledge | Provides elementary background knowledge at starting level 1pt | Gives a correct overview of the background knowledge at the appropriate level 2pt | Gives a correct and relevant overview of the background knowledge 3pt |
| Research question | Absent or not related to subject matter | Provides inoperable relationship with subject matter 1pt | Clear description of research question, but the relationship between introduction, research question and the expected answer is unclear 2pt | Clear description of research question, and the relationship between introduction, research question and the expected answer is unequivocal 3pt |
| Materials and Methods | Description of materials and/or methods is absent | Description of materials, protocols and equipment is incomplete 1pt | Description of materials and methods is complete and supplemented with details of own execution 2pt | |
| Results | Unclear, incomplete presentation of results | Unclear presentation of results 2pt | Complete and correct presentation of results 4pt | Complete and correct presentation of results that shows their relation 6pt |
| Discussion | Not more than a description of results | Explanation of results based on theory 2pt | Explanation of results based on correct interpretation of relevant theory, and on practical problems posed by flaws in materials and methods 4pt | Correct explanation of results based on correct interpretation of relevant theory, on practical problems posed by flaws in materials methods, and by restrictions of approach 6pt |
| Conclusion | Absent | Summary of discussion only 1pt | Obvious attempt to answer the research question 2pt | Correct answer to the research question 3pt |
| Sources | Absent | Incomplete and/or inadequate 1pt | Complete and adequate 2pt | Complete, adequate, showing own initiative 3pt |
| Grammar and style | Poor grammar and spelling | Hardly any spelling mistakes; reasonable grammar 1pt | No spelling mistakes; good grammar 2pt | Good grammar; creative use of language 3pt |

**Fig. 1.2** Example of a rubric used with a short report writing assignment. Students in their first month of the Biomedical Sciences bachelor's program have to report on a biochemical laboratory practical plus a computer modelling practical on enzymatic reactions. (Courtesy of Dr. Giel Bosman and Dr. Thom Oostendorp, Radboud University Medical Center in Nijmegen, The Netherlands)

## 1.1 What Is a Rubric?

*Courtesy of Team Communication in Science, LUMC, Leiden University, The Netherlands.*

**Rubric writing skills in internship report – CiS (communication in science) component.**

**Student name:** ………………………………… **Student number:** ……………………..
**Date:** ………………………………….

---

**Assignment:** writing of internship report

**Specific subject of assessment:** writing skills

**Course:** Communication in science

**Learning objectives:** The student:
- applies the structure used in scientific articles
- uses formal scientific register adequately in Dutch and English

| Structure |
|---|
| The report is appropriately organized, following conventions and allowing uninterrupted reading, including:<br>- Follows Introduction, Methods, Results & Discussion structure<br>- Defines aims and purposes clearly<br>- Reports results effectively and provides a convincing discussion of these results<br>- Offers sufficient and appropriate detail in each section, enabling the reader to follow the story being told and its relevance for the field |
| **Use of language** |
| The language used shapes the report into a clear, engaging story that contributes to the scientific discourse:<br>- Readability: the text is cohesive; signals and transitions within and between sections are effective; the report is audience-focused<br>- Register: language is concise, impersonal and formal<br>- Accuracy: use of grammar, punctuation and syntax are appropriate and accurate |
| **Participation** |
| - The student has actively participated in the workgroup |

| Comments (strong points; areas for improvement) |
|---|
|   |

| Grade for CIS assessment of report (1–10 scale) |   |
|---|---|

**Fig. 1.3** Example of a holistic rubric used in the learning trajectory Communication in Science in the Bachelor Biomedical Sciences. (Courtesy of Team Communication in Science, LUMC, Leiden University, The Netherlands)

**Table 1.1** Purpose and application of rubrics for different stakeholders

| Stakeholder | Purpose and application of rubric |
|---|---|
| All stakeholders | - The descriptors in the rubric provide a common language to discuss the assignment and its products |
| Student | - Feed-up: rubric envisages product to aim for, transparency on criteria and expected level<br>- Feedback: descriptors in the rubric matching current performance + additional personalized feedback<br>- Feed-forward: take along feedback on current performance and from descriptors in the rubric at levels higher than current performance |
| Assessor | - Guidance how to evaluate and rate |
| Examiner / examining board | - Enhancing consistent scoring by different assessors<br>- More transparent underpinning of grades/decisions |
| Teaching colleagues in other courses | - Enhance longitudinal learning and visualize growth, using the same rubric as feedback instrument over different assignments<br>- Example for design of rubrics for own teaching and assessment purposes |
| Program management | - Instrument in quality control of assessment<br>- Instrument in enhancing learning environment for students (providing feedback, transparency) |

what will be assessed and valued through a rubric. Finally using a rubric can enhance **reliability** of the assessment as it directs what will be assessed and valued and thereby also minimizes individual rating errors (e.g. halo and horn effects, central tendency, over lenient or strictness) and inter-rater variability (Salkind & Rasmussen, 2018).

Table 1.2 shows a—non-exhaustive—overview of various kinds of assignments for which a rubric could be used. Note that use of one is not necessarily limited to a single assignment or occasion. Using the same rubric on different occasions in a curriculum by different assessors on various similar tasks can be extremely valuable, especially when the aim is to visualize development over time. Such a multitude of '*measurement points*' can offer information on the ability of a student that is much more reliable and valid than a single assessment can offer. This is one of the fundamentals in the concept of programmatic assessment (Van der Vleuten & Schuwirth, 2005).

**Table 1.2** (Non-exhaustive) Overview of various kinds of assignments for which a rubric could be used

| Type | Remark |
| --- | --- |
| Written report, essay | Rubrics can be used to assess both content and writing skills. |
| Other products: Poster, website, video, etc. | If students may freely choose a medium, rubric criteria that focus on function(ality) instead of form(at) may be required |
| Oral presentation | Assessed during presentation (live observation), or afterwards (recording) |
| Portfolio | Most portfolios are non-standardized, requiring a rubric that allows flexibility |
| Oral examination | Defense of a report or project, assessment of problem-solving ability for some domain, etc. |
| Performance during:<br>- Practical sessions (laboratory, computer, excursions, internship)<br>- Psycho-motor skills (in OSCEs for example)<br>- Attitude<br>- Competence domains, such as collaboration skills, communication skills, etc. | Demonstrated in real-life situations or simulations. Assessed through direct observation or video recording |

## 1.2 Checklist for Designing a Rubric

### 1.2.1 Types of Rubric

When designing a rubric, a first choice to make is whether you want to use a holistic or analytical rubric. In a holistic rubric (see Fig. 1.3) several different criteria are taken together to evaluate the product or the behaviour as a whole. There is typically no sub-scoring per criterion; the evaluation on the rubric results in a single score corresponding to the final mark or qualification. A holistic rubric is best suited when the quality of the product as a whole cannot be well represented by the sum of its components (represented by different criteria).

In an analytical rubric (like the example in Fig. 1.2) different criteria are evaluated separately. This provides a student with more detailed feedback and allows for scoring per criterion. A next choice to be made is how to go from scores to grades (see Sect. 1.2.6). The rubric can specify a number of points in each cell, leading to a sum score that can be used to calculate the final mark or qualification. Or the assessor makes an overall decision on the mark or qualification and uses the rubric only as a guidance for feedback and underpinning of the decision (see Sect. 1.2.6).

### 1.2.2 Criteria

The evaluation criteria in a rubric should align with the learning outcomes of the learning activity being assessed. And, consistent with another rule of constructive alignment (Biggs, 1996), the learning activities should help students to achieve the learning outcomes. A common pitfall is to turn every aspect that can be observed in a product into a criterion, resulting in many different criteria. This may not only be impractical and time-consuming for assessors using the rubric, but may also impair its feedback function. For feedback to be effective (Hattie & Timperley, 2007), it is better to be sparse and focus on aspects that (1) are most relevant for this specific assignment and (2) for which students will have the opportunity to apply in another or adapted product soon. It's also important to consider the setting in which the rubric will be used. For instance, a presentation a rubric with 3–5 criteria would be more workable than one with 10 different criteria to evaluate while listening.

## 1.2.3 Rating Scale

To choose a rating scale that represents the different levels of achievement in your rubric, you should start with the purpose of the assignment and its place in your assessment strategy. For each level you need descriptors whose differences are relevant to the product or behaviour and learning outcomes to assess; avoid filling cells just to fit a scale. Our advice is to make the scale no more fine-grained than needed, as it will hamper usability of the rubric, just like too many different criteria do. Note also that there is no need to have in your rubric the same scale as used for the assignments final mark or qualification. A score based on the rubric can be transformed to any other grading scale through calculation or based on a grade conversion table. As a rule of thumb a scale with 3–5 points will suffice for most purposes and criteria. Requirements that need to be met before a product can be evaluated properly (like required format, length, the elements that need to be included, etc.) are best left out of the rubric scoring process. Either use such requirements as a check whether a product is applicable for evaluation or define them as a 'knock-out' score on the criteria in the rubric that directly leads to a fail in case of a summative assessment, no matter what score is obtained for other criteria. In both cases, resubmission of an adapted product may be the action required from students (or remediation on a next occasion). See for example the rubric in Fig. 1.2 where knock-out criteria are used as the lowest level of the scale.

## 1.2.4 Performance Descriptors

Now comes the hard but rewarding part: defining the performance descriptors in each cell of the rubric. A rubric is intended to make what is valued explicit; therefore specific language is required to '*translate*' what an experienced assessor had in mind to a description that is understandable for students. If descriptors indicate different performance levels on a criterion through general qualifications—such as 'insufficient' versus 'good' or 'excellent'—the format of a rubric is no more informative than the criteria and a rating scale. On the other hand, trying to define every single detail by which the performance on different levels differs could easily lead to clouding the most relevant aspects (feedback!) and making the rubric a tedious instrument to work with. And if for some criterion it is unrealistic to discern at all levels of the scale, it may be better to combine two levels instead of describing irrelevant differences (see for example Fig. 1.2). There are no general rules to be given. It is best to make a first draft of the rubric, together with colleague assessors, try it out on existing products or observations, and adapt where needed. Discussing with colleague assessors and students what makes a product or performance sufficient for the criterion often helps in defining the essential parts that can be taken up in the rubric cell. Usually it takes a few rounds of using, evaluating and improving before you have a rubric that fully fits the needs of the assessors and the students.

## 1.2.5 Feedback

One of the most important needs is, ultimately, to enhance learning. To meet this need we have to integrate rubrics in educational practice in such a way that rubrics support learning. As mentioned earlier rubrics can play a large role in providing feedback for students. Therefore it is worthwhile to first look at the subject of feedback in some more detail.

Although feedback in itself has a limited effect, it shows its power when students are able to use the given feedback to adapt misinterpretations and improve performance. Feedback flourishes when it is used to bridge the gap from the point of what is understood and/or mastered (pre-knowledge/competence level) and what has to be understood and/or mastered (nearby future learning objectives) (Brooks et al., 2019). Meta-analyses (Hattie & Timperley, 2007) conducted in order to search for effective strategies to enhance learning show that feedback-related activities score high on effect sizes. There are however some restrictions to consider because the effect sizes vary considerably. This means that there are ways to integrate feedback in the curriculum that enhance learning positively, but also some that do so negatively. Aspects that show positive results are practices where feedback is characterized as shown in the box below (Hattie & Timperley, 2007).

| Characteristics of feedback that have shown positive results on learning [a] |
|---|
| • Poses low threat on self-esteem |
| • Connects to earlier learning |
| • Consists of information about progress and how to proceed |
| • Presents and results in (stimulating) learning possibilities such as enhanced challenges, more self-regulation, more strategies, rather than on just the need to learn more |
| • Is given on the task, processing of the task and on self-regulation rather than on the self or personal level (usually through praise) |
| • Is provided in written comments rather than in a grade |
| • Is combined with effective instruction in the classroom |

[a] Derived from Hattie and Timperley (2007)

The diverseness of feedback is shown by various other contextual aspects one has to take into account when putting feedback into educational practice. Firstly the actors: feedback can be given by teachers, peers or external experts. Secondly the way it is transmitted: orally or written. Thirdly if it is presented qualitative and/or quantitative. Finally the aspect of ownership: there is supply-driven feedback (initiated by the teacher) versus demand-driven feedback (initiated by the student). Some experts stress the importance of student initiative where students first ask for feedback specifically before it is given, thereby taking responsibility for their own learning, and in doing so become feedback seekers (Deci & Ryan, 1985). This insight can be valuable information when integrating rubrics in daily practice in order to introduce learning activities around rubrics that also stimulate students to take initiative by seeking feedback rather than only passively receiving it in preparation for an upcoming assessment.

Based on literature and effect sizes of practices, Hattie and Timperley (2007) suggest a model how to integrate feedback in learning along three main questions which the learner needs to address:

1. Where am I going? (feed-up)
2. How am I doing? (feedback)
3. What next? (feed-forward)

Given these insights the question remains how to integrate rubrics in such a way that it enhances learning through the use of feedback. In Table 1.3 we show an example. The activities shown in this example can be considered as 'modular elements' that can be used or not, depending on your vision, the context of your lessons and practical considerations.

## 1.2.6 Marking, Scores, Norms and Grades

Note that in the example in Table 1.3 the element of grading is also incorporated as a part of feedback. Of course it can be considered as such, although it is a rather limited input to enhance learning. Nevertheless grades are an important extrinsic motivational element for students. Often to the dismay of many teachers, students ask: 'Do we need to learn this for our exam?' We might not like questions like this but it is an important one for teachers, students and faculty. Several studies show that students value rubrics because of the transparency in grading that is given by the teacher. This motivates them and gives them more understanding of the reason of the given grade (Andrade et al., 2010). With scoring, the question of reliability is an important one. In most of the studies it appears that teachers assess more consistent, objective and more efficiently while using rubrics (Andrade et al., 2010). Nevertheless contextual factors do influence this, such as the quality of the rubric. Furthermore there are other aspects that can enhance reliability. Firstly the number of assessors that grade an assignment. Two or more assessors grading the same

## 1.2 Checklist for Designing a Rubric

**Table 1.3** Example of a course where rubrics are integrated in order to enhance feedback and learning

| TEACHER ACTIVITIES | SELECTION OF ACTIVITIES IN THE FEEDBACK LOOP | STUDENT ACTIVITIES |
|---|---|---|
| **How do I connect to the knowledge base?** | **1. Feed up** | **What am I going to do?** |
| Constructing the rubric with students | Workgroups | Co-authoring the rubric |
| Handing over the rubric to students | Digital learning environment | Studying the rubric in preparing for the assignment |
| **How do I check the level of my students?** | **2. Feedback** | **How am I doing?** |
| Monitoring asked, given and received peer review | Online peer review on product and/or process | Asking, giving and receiving peer review based on rubric |
| Discussing product/process and peer review with students | Progress monitoring talks | Discussing product/process and peer review with students and teachers |
| Giving feedback and grading with the rubric | Assessment | Students submit product(s) |
| **What does the student need for further development?** | **3. Feed-forward** | **What will be my next steps?** |
| Discussing feedback and given grade and assisting in formulating new learning goals with rubric as reference | Ending the course and preparing for the next | Students ask questions after receiving grade and feedback and formulate new learning goals with rubric as reference |

assignment instead of one has a positive effect on reliability of the score. Secondly reliability can be improved in the design of the rubrics. It is recommended to use earlier student work to describe the different levels and to first test a rubric with the assessors involved. Altogether it is worthwhile to acknowledge that assessing behaviour in assignments of tasks or assessing products does always have a more subjective character compared to a written knowledge exam with closed response formats like multiple-choice questions. The use of rubrics though supports valid assessment types such as self-, co- and peer assessment as well as portfolio assessments. Note the word *supports* is used here: rubrics should not be seen as a recipe in which the sum of sub-scores of all criteria leads to a 100% reliable total score. When assessing competences it seems important to lower expectancies of the reliability of one assessment and consider the use of more than one moment to assess to increase reliability (Schuwirth & van der Vleuten, 2012). Overall there is a tendency to use rubrics more when grading. This is probably because of the lack of alternatives for teachers: grading with rubrics objectivates the assessment more than grading with no external guidance.

When we look at the actual grading of the scores, experts say that this should be a logical process rather than a mathematical process. This means that scoring 3 out of 6 points should not automatically lead to 50% of the total grade (Mertler, 2000). In practice using rubric scores this way might be one of the reasons of often heard frustration with assessors when they feel that they do not always agree with the grade after assessing with the rubric. This frustration can be overcome by weighing the different criteria and thereby rewarding the most essential criteria with more points. The cut-off score that discerns a pass from a fail should be a decision of the teacher and his/her colleagues. Ultimately they are the ones that are able to weigh the different criteria proportionally, reflecting their knowledge of the discipline and the challenge some criteria pose students to meet them.

So the weighing of criteria and position of cut-off score should be taken into account in the design of a scoring rubric. The enclosure of a so-called qualitative comments field, in addition to the descriptors in the rubric, seems a solid improvement as well. Especially considering the fact that it is almost impossible and not desirable to pre-describe all possible behaviours in an assignment, the overload of information would only lead to confusion and hamper usability of the rubric. By describing specifics of the actual behaviour and interpreting this behaviour, such qualitative comments will increase satisfaction with the given grade for teachers and students. It contributes to a better reflection of the actual observed behaviour, which might not always be the case in detailed pre-described rubrics without these qualitative remarks/feedback.

## 1.3 How to Use a Rubric?

### 1.3.1 The Assessment Process: Choices to Be Made

In addition to choices regarding the design of the rubric, discussed above, there are several choices to be made on how to use the rubric in your assessment process. These are summarized in Table 1.4.

Some additional explanation regarding timing of distribution of the rubric is in place. Making the rubric available to students at the start of the assignment probably serves student learning best. This might seem somewhat counter-intuitive, as a rubric has to do with evaluation and assessment that is often seen as a conclusive part of education. However, as explained in Sect. 1.1.2 we plea to stimulate students to use the rubrics themselves, so the tasks ahead for them are clearer and they gradually learn to evaluate their own performance.

## 1.3 How to Use a Rubric?

**Table 1.4** Summary of procedural choices to make when using a rubric

| Choice | Options | Examples and remarks |
|---|---|---|
| **Purpose of use** | Formative feedback and/or summative assessment? | |
| | Evaluating current performance or focusing on growth compared to a previous performance? | |
| **Distribution** | Medium: Rubric on paper or digital? | LMS and other educational software often include functionality to build-in your rubric, facilitate the scoring process, add extra written feedback, and communicate results to students. Digitizing your rubric has also the advantage that scores can automatically be stored, facilitating evaluation (described in Sect. 1.3.2). |
| | Timing: At the start of and during the assignment instead of only afterwards as feedback with the scoring results (we highly recommend this as explained above) | |
| **Link to learning activities** | Although a rubric can just be made available to students, it could also be used in teaching activities in many different ways to provide extra learning opportunities either before, during or after working on the assignment | - Evaluate some example products together with students<br>- Discuss what students think defines an excellent, good or insufficient performance and use this to design or adjust descriptors or weighing of criteria in the rubric<br>- Student self-assessment with peer and/or teacher assessment and discuss any major differences<br>- Supervisor shares general findings like frequently occurring flaws and common misunderstandings, offering extra explanation or practice regarding criteria that students in general had most difficulty with |
| **Marking** | What to mark?<br>Product/performance and criteria need to be aligned with learning outcomes and teaching activities | This is part of rubric design (see Sect. 1.2) |
| | How to mark?<br>Analytical or holistic scoring.<br>Define soring scale and — if applicable— choice of cut-off score and grading | This is part of rubric design (see Sect. 1.2) |
| | Who marks?<br>Students (self- and/or peer assessment supervisors and/or others<br>Number of assessors, 1 or more | Others could for example be the client or patient in a simulation or real-life setting |
| | When to mark?<br>Only at the end of the assignment, evaluating the final product or performance?<br>Or also intermediate? | Reasons for intermediate use: For instance as formative feedback to improve the final product or performance (e.g. peer feedback on collaboration skills half-way during a group assignment, or formative feedback of peers and/or supervisors on (some paragraphs of) a draft report) |

**Tab. 1.4** (continued)

|  |  | Furthermore, evaluation of an essential intermediate step in the assignment could be required when it may not be observable any more in the end product (e.g. in dentistry the drill hole before filling a tooth) and/or in case errors have to be amended to allow continuing the assignment (e.g. some programming code or settings in a modelling assignment or lab experiment) |
|---|---|---|

## *1.3.2 Evaluation and Improvement*

You designed your rubric and put it into practice. But how do you evaluate the results? Practices and parameters that you may be familiar with in the context of other (written) examination can be helpful for the evaluation of an assignment that uses a rubric. These are summarized in Table 1.5.

Evaluating a combination of such parameters is an excellent means to improve your rubric. Like the development of the rubric, involve your colleague assessors and possibly students in the improvement process. Improvement is likely to focus on the way performance descriptors are formulated and arranging them to the appropriate level. Skipping or adding criteria or changing the weighing of criteria will probably improve the rubric as well. Test the adapted rubric again on some existing product before you put it into practice again.

Furthermore, evaluation results can help you to improve procedures for using the rubric, both for students and assessors. Instructions can be improved, for example to include an additional requirement that needs to be met before handing in the assignment. If the rubric scores indicate a criterion was very difficult for students, the instruction or assignment itself can be adapted, or prior learning activities may be added or adapted to help students master some extra knowledge or skill required.

As already mentioned before it usually takes some rounds of using, evaluating and improving before you have a rubric that fully fits the needs of the assessors and the students.

Table 1.5 Summary of parameters to evaluate a rubric

| Parameter | What to look for | Remarks |
|---|---|---|
| **Score distribution: mean, variance, range** | Difficulty: what percentages of the maximum score did students receive? Discrimination: what is the difference between highest and lowest scores? Check also for the scoring per criterion. Consistency: was some criterion very difficult or easy compared to others? And if so, is this criterion indeed testing a different ability? If not, check if the descriptors for this criterion are adequate and on the right level | If possible, also compare with scores that other students got previously on the same assignment |
| **Coherence** | Do results correlate with students other assessment information? And if not, is this assignment and rubric indeed testing a different ability? | Focus on assessments of similar tasks / learning outcomes. Comparison with results obtained through different assessment methods may strengthen your validity argument |
| **Inter-rater variance** | If each product/performance is assessed by multiple raters, calculate inter-rater reliability. If single raters apply, compare score distribution between raters: is there any systematically high scorer (dove) or low scorer (hawk)? | Agreement after dialogue, or valid different views? Prohibitive differences: consider re-assessing a sample of the products to calibrate scores |
| **Student evaluation** | Clear, transparent, acknowledgement and acceptance of resulting scores? Useful for feed-up, feed back, feed-forward? Suitable for self-assessment? Actual use (timing, aim, experience)? Suggestions for improvement? | Consider adapting the rubric, the assignment or its instructions for students, and possibly provide some extra teaching activity or materials |
| **Assessor evaluation** | Clear, acknowledgement and acceptance of resulting scores? Experiences while using? Suggestions for improvement? | Consider adapting the rubric, the assignment or its instructions for assessors, and plan a kick-of/calibration session with assessors before applying again |

# References

Andrade, H. L., Du, Y., & Mycek, K. (2010). Rubric-referenced self-assessment and middle school students' writing. *Assessment in Education: Principles, Policy & Practice, 17*(2), 199–214.

Biggs, J. (1996). Enhancing teaching through constructive alignment. *Higher Education, 32*(3), 347–364.

Brooks, C., Carroll, A., Gillies, R. M., & Hattie, J. (2019). A matrix of feedback for learning. *Australian Journal of Teacher Education, 44*(4).

Deci, E. L., & Ryan, R. M. (1985). *Intrinsic motivation and self-determination in human behavior*. Plenum.

Garrison, D. R. (1997). Self-directed learning: Toward a comprehensive model. *Adult Education Quarterly, 48*(1), 18–33.

Hattie, J., & Timperley, H. (2007). The power of feedback. *Review of Educational Research, 77*(1), 81–112.

Martinez, M. E., & Lipson, J. I. (1989). Assessment for learning. *Educational Leadership, 47*, 73–75.

Mertler, C. A. (2000). Designing scoring rubrics for your classroom. *Practical Assessment, Research, and Evaluation, 7*, 25.

Reddy, Y. M., & Andrade, H. (2010). A review of rubric use in higher education. *Assessment & Evaluation in Higher Education, 35*(4), 435–448.

Salkind, N. J., & Rasmussen, K. (Eds.). (2018). *Encyclopedia of educational psychology*. Sage Publications.

Schuwirth, L. W. T., & van der Vleuten, C. P. M. (2012). Programmatic assessment and Kane's validity perspective. *Medical Education, 46*(1), 38–48.

Stevens, D., & Levi, A. J. (2013). *Introduction to rubrics: An assessment tool to save grading time, convey effective feedback, and promote student learning*. Stylus Publishing.

van der Vleuten, C. P. M., & Schuwirth, L. W. T. (2005). Assessing professional competence: From methods to programmes. *Medical Education, 39*, 309–317.

# Chapter 2
# Rubrics: Best Practices

## Contents

| | | |
|---|---|---|
| 2.1 | Rubric for a Written Assignment. | 18 |
| | 2.1.1 Context in Which the Rubric Is Developed and Used. | 18 |
| | 2.1.2 Construction of the Rubric for a Written Assignment. | 19 |
| | 2.1.3 Use of the Rubric in Practice. | 21 |
| 2.2 | Rubric for an Oral Presentation. | 22 |
| | 2.2.1 Context in Which the Rubric Is Developed and Used. | 23 |
| | 2.2.2 Construction of the Rubric for an Oral Presentation. | 23 |
| | 2.2.3 Use of the Rubric in Practice. | 25 |
| 2.3 | Rubric for Collaboration Skills. | 29 |
| | 2.3.1 Context in Which the Rubric Is Developed and Used. | 29 |
| | 2.3.2 Construction of the Rubric for Collaboration Skills. | 30 |
| | 2.3.3 Use of the Rubric in Practice. | 30 |
| 2.4 | Rubric for Clinical Skills. | 31 |
| | 2.4.1 Context in Which the Rubric Is Developed and Used. | 35 |
| | 2.4.2 Construction of the Rubric to Assess Clinical Skills. | 35 |
| | 2.4.3 Use of the Rubrics in Practice. | 39 |
| References. | | 40 |

**Abstract** In this chapter we describe four best practices of using rubrics for assessment and feedback, in different educational settings and for various teaching activities. We describe a rubric for a written assignment, for an oral presentation, for collaboration skills and for clinical skills and how to use these in practice. For each of these best practices first the educational setting and context is portrayed. Then the process of construction of the rubric is described: the criteria for assessment, the rating scale and the performance descriptors. We also describe the communication processes with other teachers involved and students. Finally the use of the rubric in clinical and biomedical teaching practice is described in more detail: how the grading, assessment and feedback are organized, and how the rubrics and procedures evolve through evaluation and experience.

## 2.1 Rubric for a Written Assignment

| Rubric | Written assignments, scientific reporting |
|---|---|
| Educational program | Bachelor Biomedical Sciences |
| Faculty | Radboud University Medical Center |
| University | Radboud University, Nijmegen, The Netherlands |
| Course | Associations and causal relations–Research your own data (RYOD) |
| Course coordinator | Dr. F. de Vegt |
| Written by | Dr. F. de Vegt (associate professor of Epidemiology education at Radboudumc) |

### 2.1.1 Context in Which the Rubric Is Developed and Used

'*Research*' is one of the longitudinal tracks in the Biomedical Sciences bachelors' program at Radboud University Nijmegen since 2015. In this track, students learn biomedical research methods, ranging from laboratory skills and performing physical measurements to data management and statistical analyses. In addition, they learn how to present and communicate research findings, by practicing with scientific writing and oral presentation.

In our practice-based learning approach, first-year students are actively involved in biomedical research by collecting data from themselves and their peers. After obtaining informed consent, in the first three quartiles students measure and collect data concerning anthropometry, heart rate variability and other ECG findings and food consumption. They also collect a morning urine sample for biochemical analyses (such as urea, creatinine and pH). In addition, students are asked to fill out the SQUASH questionnaire on physical activity (Wendel-Vos et al., 2003; Campbell et al., 2016) and a questionnaire on lifestyle habits. In a lab class students isolate DNA from saliva, and use standard genetic lab techniques (PRC and Sanger sequencing) to measure four different genetic variants in their DNA. In addition they measure four common traits that are known to be associated with these genotypes (Eriksson et al., 2010). In all quartiles, students practice with data analyses and writing scientific reports concerning the specific data collection and measurements. These reports follow the editorial requirements of scientific papers, like abstracts, introduction, methods, results and discussion.

During the first year, all data are entered and merged into one student research database. In the last quartile of the year, all biomedical students get access to the (anonymous) database. They formulate a research question of their own choice, perform the statistical data analyses and write a short research paper (Assignment 'Research Your Own Data', RYOD). This RYOD research paper focuses on the description of the methods and results, specifically the use of tables and figures. The research papers are assessed using a rubric by experienced researchers who also

## 2.1 Rubric for a Written Assignment

give additional narrative feedback on the students' research reports. This 'research your own data' approach and the appreciation by students have been described in more detail elsewhere (de Vegt et al., 2021).

### 2.1.2 Construction of the Rubric for a Written Assignment

**Setting Criteria (*Rubric Rows*)** The first rubric for the 'Research Your Own Data' (RYOD) written assignment was developed in 2015, and during the years thereafter it has been adjusted and evolved into the rubric as it is currently used (Fig. 2.1). There are 14 criteria in total, of which 12 are related to scientific content and resemble major requirements for scientific papers (such as *'describe the study design'* and *'figures'*). Criteria 13 and 14 are related to general structure, use of scientific language, grammar and layout.

**Rating Scale (*Rubric Columns*)** The rating scale is described in four columns and goes from '*insufficient, needs rewriting*' to '*excellent*'. This rating scale is used for all written assignments in the research longitudinal track in the bachelor's degree program Biomedical Sciences. The third column *'sufficient/good'* is the expected level, which should correspondent with a grade 7–7.5 (scale 1–10). The first column *'insufficient, needs rewriting'* is only used when for a particular assignment a criterion is very important and that part in the report should be rewritten when insufficient. For some criteria two rating columns are merged, for example for study design (merging of *'sufficient/good'* and *'excellent'*), as no clear distinction can be made in the description and requirements.

**Performance Descriptors (*Rubric Cells*)** In the cells the desirable performance is described for each criterion and rating scale. The cells describe in words the expected level a student needs to achieve, which is directly related to the end product (in this case a written scientific report). The process of making these descriptions is very important and time-consuming and requires a lot of consultation with other teachers involved and educational advisors. Scores are also assigned to each cell, making it possible to calculate grades for the total assignment based on a sum score. Certain criteria may be counting heavier than others, for example, the criterion *'data collection'* scores from 0 to 6, while *'layout and general structure'* scores from 1 to 4.

**Construction and Fine-Tuning with Other Teachers** Every year the rubric is fine-tuned and small adjustments are made, based on the experience of the last year cycle of teaching the course and the grading and feedback round of the written reports. All teachers involved in grading the report may suggest changes for the rubric and the process of grading. Before the next edition of the course starts, all teachers will receive the final, updated version of the rubric.

| | Insufficient, needs rewriting | Deficient, can be compensated | Sufficient/good | Excellent |
|---|---|---|---|---|
| 1. Title | | Title does not match content 1 | Title provides sufficient information on content 3 | Title is appealing and provides clear information on content and main conclusions 4 |
| 2. Research question | Absent or incorrect 0 | (set of) Research questions are incomplete or formulation may be improved 2 | Correctly formulated as a researchable (set of) questions 4 | Attractively and clearly formulated as a researchable (set of) questions, complete, unambiguous, singular and relevant 6 |
| 3. Study population | Absent 0 | Insufficient description of study population 2 | Sufficient and correct description of the study population 4 | Excellent description of the study population (clear, correct and concise) 6 |
| 4. Study design | | Insufficiently described / wrong study design 1 | Clearly described and correct study design 3 | |
| 5. Data collection | Absent 0 | Basic, incomplete or incorrect description of data collection / measurements 2 | Sufficient description of methods of data collection and data handling 4 | Excellent and clear description of methods of data collection and handling 6 |
| 6. Statistical analysis | Absent 0 | Basic, incomplete or incorrect description or choice of statistical techniques 2 | Correct choice and sufficient and correct description of statistical techniques 4 | Clear, complete and correct description of data analysis. Correct choice of statistical techniques 6 |
| 7. Results–text | Absent 0 | Basic, incomplete or unclear description of results 2 | Sufficient and correct description of results 4 | Complete, correct and clear description of results 6 |
| 8. Results–tables | No tables, or a table with non-relevant data, or table is a copy of SPSS output 0 | Tables with relevant results 2 | Tables with relevant results, mostly complete with title, legend and proper formatting of content 4 | Tables with relevant results, clear and complete with title, legend and proper formatting of content and in support of the text 6 |
| 9. Results–figures | No figure 0 | Figures with relevant results 2 | Figures with relevant results, mostly complete with title, legend and proper axis 4 | Figures with relevant results, clear and complete with title, legend and proper axis and in support of the text 6 |
| 10. Results–statistical test | | No statistical test performed, or statistical test is incorrect or without clear interpretation 1 | Statistical test performed correctly and with a sufficient and clear interpretation 4 | |
| 11. Discussion | Absent 0 | Insufficient description of two strong and two weak points of the study 2 | Sufficient and clear description of two strong and two weak points of the study 5 | Excellent description of the two strong and weak points of the study, with some suggestions for improvement 7 |
| 12. Conclusion | | No conclusion or conclusion is unclear 1 | Sufficient and clear conclusion 3 | Clear conclusion which answers the research question 5 |
| 13. Use of scientific language and grammar | | Poor use of scientific language. Poor grammar and spelling 2 | Sufficient use of scientific language. Hardly any spelling mistakes; reasonable grammar 4 | No spelling mistakes; good grammar; creative use of scientific language. Attractive to read. 6 |
| 14. Layout and general structure | | Layout is sufficient, but lacks consistency. No or incorrect headings 1 | Clear layout and structure (readable font, use of headings and proper style of formatting) 4 | |

**Fig. 2.1** Rubric for the 'Research Your Own Data' (RYOD) written assignment

## 2.1 Rubric for a Written Assignment

**Communication to Students** All course materials are placed at Brightspace, a cloud-based learning management system (Brightspace, D2L Corporation, n.d.). Students are informed before the start of the course about the learning goals of the course and the criteria for assessment including the rubric.

### 2.1.3 Use of the Rubric in Practice

During the '*Research your own data*' (RYOD) course, students learn how to develop their own research question by using the student research database. They also learn how to do the statistical analyses by using statistical software. The students then have to write their scientific report individually, focusing on the research question, the description of the methods, and the results in text, tables and figures. The students have to upload their report in Brightspace, the learning management system (Brightspace, D2L Corporation, n.d.).

**Grading and Feedback** For the grading and feedback process using the rubric, the program Turn-it-in is used (Turn-it-in, n.d., Turnitin.com). Turn-it-in is an integrated tool in Brightspace with a rubric function. In addition, reports can be checked for plagiarism by Turn-it-in. The RYOD rubric is uploaded in the program and used for the grading. The assessor assigns for all criteria the appropriate score, and the total score is calculated by the program (Fig. 2.2). The maximum score in the RYOD rubric is 75 points. The total count in the column '*sufficient/good*', which is the expected level, is 54 (72% of the maximum score). For a sufficient final grade a student should have at least 42 points (absolute pass mark 55%). If a student has a 0 score for a criterion, the final grade will be insufficient (independent of the total score) and the report needs to be (partly) rewritten.

Besides the score, extra feedback is given as 'written comments' also in Turn-it-in. The assessor can indicate to which criterion the comment belongs, but also general feedback may be given. Frequently given feedback can be saved as a 'quick mark' that can be re-used, making it more easier and faster to provide this feedback to many students.

**Evaluation and Improvement** In this RYOD assignment, we have a team of 5 or 6 assessors to grade the near 100 individually written scientific reports. For the alignment, all assessors first grade two reports, and they will discuss the assessment of these reports. Then the criteria and how to use them in practice are clear to everyone, and the grading process of all reports can start. All assessors communicate their grading and questions about grading with the examiner (FdV), who has the final responsibility for the grading process. This examiner checks some grades and feedback to improve equality in the grading process between the team of assessors. After the grading process, a short report with the range and mean final grades is sent to the team assessors. This report also includes general remarks and findings from the grading and feedback process.

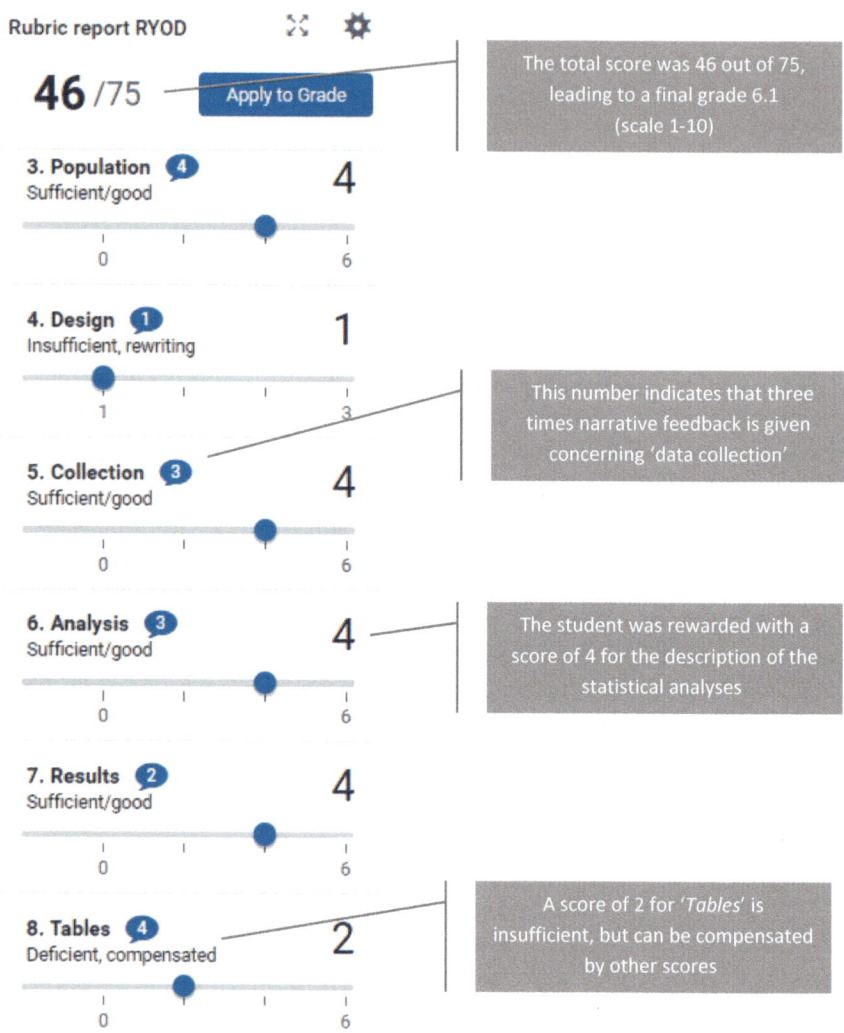

**Fig. 2.2** Scores to the criteria in the RYOD rubric. (Turnitin.com)

## 2.2 Rubric for an Oral Presentation

| | |
|---|---|
| Rubric | Scientific oral presentation |
| Educational program | Bachelor Biomedical Sciences |
| Faculty | Leiden University Medical Center (LUMC) |
| University | Leiden University, Leiden, The Netherlands |
| Course | Start.BW: introduction in biomedical thinking |
| Course coordinator | Dr. N.A. Gruis (associate professor at LUMC) |
| Written by | Drs. I. de Boer (educational advisor at LUMC) |

## 2.2.1 Context in Which the Rubric Is Developed and Used

The 3 years program of the Bachelor Biomedical Sciences at the University of Leiden hosts about 70 students per year. The first course in the first year is called *'Start.BW: introduction in biomedical thinking'*. This short 2-week course is all about laying the fundaments and further uplifting enthusiasm for what is to come in a research-intensive program. In the course students are introduced to one of many topics in the biomedical field: the challenges faced as a result of the skin cancer epidemic. At the end of the course students present in pairs their most important research findings by (partially) answering one of the major research questions on this topic. In order to do so they learn basic biomedical concepts related to skin cancer, to systematically conduct a literature search, how to answer a research question and orally report on this in a scientific manner. A rubric is used to grade a scientific oral presentation in which students present their findings (answers) to a research question. The rubric is also used by the teachers to guide students during their work on the research questions and their preparation of the oral presentation.

The initial incentive for the construction of the rubric was twofold: firstly the desire to have a framework in order to substantiate the given grades and lower subjectivity of given grades. Secondly to better guide students in their development of the required skills during the course. The idea was that students could use the rubric also in following courses when presenting research findings in another biomedical context, thus forming a learning trajectory throughout the program. This was envisioned from the notion that being able to give a scientific presentation is a skill that takes some time and practice to master. Other course coordinators were therefore stimulated to use the rubric as well. Integration of the rubric in the existing learning trajectories 'communication in science' or 'biomedical and scientific training' could be a next step.

## 2.2.2 Construction of the Rubric for an Oral Presentation

**Setting Criteria (*Rubric Rows*)** One of the first steps in constructing the rubric (see Fig. 2.3) several years ago was the selection of the criteria, this being the rows in the rubric. It was already clear at that time that the focus in the course lay on students being able to present their findings in a scientific manner rather than developing mere presentation skills.

With the course objectives in mind, the answer to the following questions leads to the criteria (rows) in the rubric: what do we expect students to master at the end of the course and what do we want to see in the oral presentation?

**Rating Scale (*Rubric Columns*)** After that the assessment levels (columns in the rubric) were chosen. At the start of the construction the rubric consisted of four levels but gradually three levels were preferred. Reason for this was that it proved

| Criterion | Below level (1 point) | On level (2 points) | Above level (3 points) |
|---|---|---|---|
| The title and introduction… | show partially the main subject itself and its relevance. | show the main subject and its relevance. | show the main subject and its relevance and serves to introduce the research question. |
| The research question / goal … | follows does not follow logically after the introduction | is clear, fits the title and introduction. May be a bit wide / broad; May be formulated somewhat broad. | Is clear, fits the title and introduction and is well specified. |
| The results… | are mentioned, but visual support such as graphics and tables, figures is not given on places where needed. | are clear and visual supportive tables, graphics and figures support the main message. | are clear and visual supportive tables, graphics and figures are well chosen and support the main message logically. |
| The discussion… | lacks depth, misses crucial information and insufficiently shows the main message or aspects. | has sufficient depth and shows important aspects. | Shows depth, all main aspects discussed in detail and shows a critical review. |
| The conclusion… | gives no clear answer on the research question. | gives a clear answer to the research question. | Gives a clear and well balanced answer to the research question and gives suggestions for further research. |
| The structure (title, research question, material and methods, results, discussion, conclusion) of the presentation… | is not balanced and/or lacks aspects. | is there but not necessarily in a balanced way. | is there and in a good balance. |
| Placing the research in a scientific field/domain/theory… | is done briefly and not sufficiently backed with relevant scientific information from articles, websites or books. | is sufficiently backed with relevant scientific information from articles, websites or books. | is elaborately backed with high quality scientific information from articles, website or books. |
| The communication of information… | does not fit the target audience, is too simple or too complicated. | partially fits the target audience, is on some points too simple or too complicated. | fits the target audience, illustrates / explains and leaves out illustration / explanation where necessary. |
| The references to the sources of information… | are incomplete making it impossible to trace all information sources. | are complete, making it possible to trace all information sources. | are mentioned according to scientific conventions. |
| Content of scientific presentation… | is minimal. Introduction, research question, analysis and interpretation are not coherent and/or lack clarity. | is sufficient. Introduction, research question, analysis and interpretation are coherent and clear. | is good. Introduction, research question and analysis are clear and relevant. Interpretation and discussion are excellent. |

**Fig. 2.3** Rubric for an oral presentation on communicating scientific research

difficult to formulate four levels that were all considered meaningful and mutually distinctive. The insufficient level for instance often was described as *'not there'* or *'missing'* and this was considered unrealistic. It also became clear that for some criteria four levels could be formulated but for other criteria four levels could not be described without formulating in vague or rather subjective terms.

**Performance Descriptors (*Rubric Cells*)** The central idea behind describing the cells in the rubric was first and foremost the notion that preferably all or at least most of the descriptions should be observable for the assessors. For most of the criteria the cells in the columns *'on level'* were described first, thus answering the question: *'what is our minimum level considered sufficient?'* This, besides downsizing the amount of levels to three, helped the constructors a lot to formulate clearer, more observable and better assessable descriptions of the desired results in the cells at each level.

**Construction and Fine-Tuning with Other Teachers** Initial construction of the rubric was done by the course coordinator who is also a teacher in the course together with educational advisors. The rubric is evaluated each year. At the end of each course, teachers (tutors and assessors) discuss suggestions with the course coordinator. This has led to some changes in the descriptions of the cells over the years. Each year the latest version of the rubric is sent to the teachers together with information regarding the steps assessors need to take before (reading the rubric, using it in guiding the students during the preparation phase) and during the assessment itself.

**Communication to Students** Students find the rubric initially at the start of the course in their digital learning environment with all other course documents. The rubric is then used in the teaching activities of the workgroup teacher who guides the students in their research activities and preparation of the oral presentation. After the assessment, the students see the filled in scores by each of the two assessors.

## 2.2.3 Use of the Rubric in Practice

All students in each workgroup prepare and present their findings in pairs. They are assessed in an oral presentation with the rubric by two assessors (the workgroup teacher who guided the students during preparation and a staff member who was not involved in guiding the students). A digital rubric has been used over the years for assessing: the assessors use a laptop or tablet when assessing the presentations. In September 2020 all education was online because of the Covid-19 pandemic. Therefore, both the final presentation and the assessment were online then: assessors could follow the live presentations at their homes or offices on their laptop and they would fill in their actual scores on a second device during and right after each presentation. The steps during assessment taken by assessors in the digital assessment program are shown in Fig. 2.4.

Selecting students:

| Cancel | TEST | | Next |
|---|---|---|---|
| Activity TEST | assessor Andries | | preview |
| Cohort BW2014 | group BW2014 WG1 | | |

Student 1:

Te|

149045 Lisette
138988 Juliette

student

Student 3:

student

☐ Show all students in the cohort

BW2014 WG1

Scoring the criteria:

| New Form | TEST |
|---|---|

**Complete your selection**

**The title and introduction...**

- ⦿ cover the main subject partially and mentions relevance partially
- ◯ cover the main subject and relevance
- ◯ cover the main subject and relevance and introduces the research question logically

**The research question / the goal...**

- ⦿ does not follow logically after the introduction
- ◯ is clear, fits the title and introduction, may be formulated somewhat broad
- ◯ is clear, fits the title and introduction, well marked out

**The results...**

- ◯ are described but visual supportive graphs, tables, figures, etc. are missing on places where needed
- ◯ are described and visual supportive graphs, tables, figures, etc. match argumentation well
- ◯ are clear and the visual supportive graphs, tables, figures, etc. are well chosen and fit the argumentation logically

**Fig. 2.4** Activities of the assessor in the self-built assessment program

**Grading and Feedback** The wish to minimize subjectivity in grading was felt a difficult task, yet looking back constructing and introducing the rubric itself has helped a lot. The assessors are instructed to base their scores on the criteria in the rubric alone. Other factors such as how assessors experienced students during preparation or the notion that the students just have started their academic education are thus left out of the assessment. In order to further minimize subjectivity it was decided that a grade would consist of an average of two grades by two assessors (thereby using the four eyes principle).

When first using the rubric, we noticed that assessors would observe a presentation and then were inclined to postpone their judgement. The longer the time lap between observation and grading, the more they were inclined to use subjective arguments for their decisions. Therefore, it was decided to use a digital rubric instead of a paper rubric, making it impossible for an assessor to change a decision or score in the program, once given. A self-build program by a staff member of the ICT & Education team is used for assessment. In the program the rubric is presented and assessors can click or point on the observed level for each of the criteria. The choice for a self-build program was made because it was considered the best option to integrate all functional wishes of the course coordinator and to make quick, tailor-made, changes in the program if needed.

Besides the grading, giving feedback with the rubric to the students was considered important. It proved however difficult to do so in detail during presentations itself because the assessors needed all their attention on observing the presentation. Besides that it was considered that students would gain the most of detailed feedback in the preparation phase of the assignment rather than at the end of the course during or right after the actual presentation. Therefore it was decided that the tutors guiding the small groups would use the rubric in their discussions with the groups during preparation (intermediate feedback). At the end it is clear from the rubric on which levels students scored and this gives students feedback at the end: they can see what they should have done to obtain a higher level as described in the rubric. In addition to their individual scores and feedback, students also "receive feedback on" how they scored in comparison to other students on all criteria (Fig. 2.5).

**Evaluation and Improvement** Each presentation is graded by at least two assessors. An important bonus of the rubric being used digitally is that the grades given by all assessors can be easily compared in the system afterwards. Some assessors seem to be harsher than others. This information can be discussed with assessors so they are aware of this in future assessments. Sometimes an assessor makes a mistake by selecting the wrong student out of a given list. This led to the habit to immediately check all given scores right after the presentations, so it can be checked immediately with the assessor. Immediate consultation with the assessors is also done when two assessors defer more than one point in grading. The two assessors can substantiate their arguments for the given grade based on the submitted presentation slides and if needed the grade is changed. This step is built in the assessment process before students receive their grade. Uniformity in scoring is further stimulated by submitting the presentation slides in the virtual learning environment before the presentations are given. By looking at the students presentation slides before the assessment, the assessors are better prepared for their upcoming task.

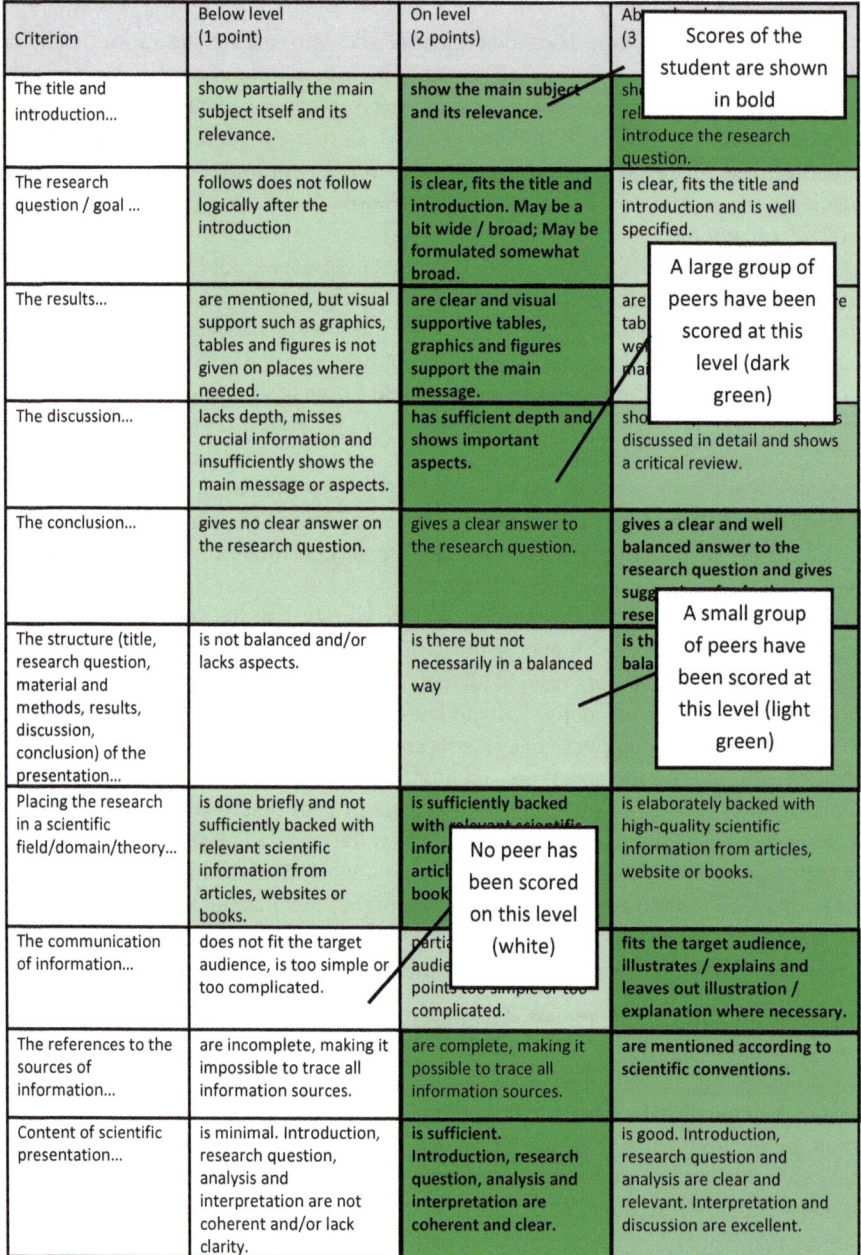

**Fig. 2.5** Results individual student and their peers shown to students in the self-built assessment program

## 2.3 Rubric for Collaboration Skills

| Rubric | For collaboration and team skills |
|---|---|
| Educational program | Bachelor Nutrition and Health (in collaboration with BSc Biology and BSc Animal Sciences) |
| University | Wageningen University and Research, the Netherlands |
| Course | Collaboration skills—learning trajectory |
| Course coordinator | Dr W.T. Steegenga—assistant professor at WU (in collaboration with skills and educational experts S. Zijlstra, MSc, MA, and Dr. J. Gulikers plus Dr M. Coppens for the Biology and Dr I. Palm for the Animal Sciences programme) |
| Written by | Dr. M. Latijnhouwers (assessment expert at WU) |

### 2.3.1 Context in Which the Rubric Is Developed and Used

Wageningen University (WU) postulated in its *Vision for Education 2017* the ambition to give non-discipline specific competences more prominence and defined '*collaboration*' as one of the required academic skills in all its academic bachelor's degree programs. For each skill a coherent and structured set of learning activities should be embedded as a visible learning trajectory in all bachelor's degree programs. In such a learning trajectory the student is offered instruction, repeated exercise, feedback (from teachers or peers) and assessment, thus taking a skill to a higher level step by step.

To illustrate the developmental path three attainment levels are discerned for all skills. The minimum level required for a bachelor's degree is at least level 2 for all the academic skills and level 1 for the reflection and learning skills. Programs set their own emphases as they choose for which of the skills students should reach a higher attainment level (mandatory for at least 70% of all the skills), depending on the specific character of their program.

For collaboration skills, a 3-year innovation project started to design, develop and implement procedures and tools for teaching, practicing and assessment. The BSc degree programs involved as pioneers in this project were Nutrition and Health, Biology, and Animal Sciences. The project team consisted of a skills coordinator for each of these programs plus educational experts of the Education and Learning Sciences department. The educationalist developed the materials in consultation with the other team members while the skills coordinator focused on integrating the whole collaboration skill learning trajectory in existing courses and skills learning activities in their program. In September 2018 the developed materials were for the first time put into practice in year 1 of the Nutrition and Health BSc program. And, after evaluation and improvement, in September 2019 they were implemented in year 1 of all three programs and year 2 of Nutrition and Health.

## 2.3.2 Construction of the Rubric for Collaboration Skills

**Setting Criteria (*Rubric Rows*)** To operationalize the general term '*collaboration*' to observable student behaviour, the developers started with defining a set of qualifications describing a successful collaborator. This way several '*micro-skills*' were defined as criteria for feedback and assessment (see Fig. 2.6).

**Rating Scale (*Rubric Columns*)** The scale of distinct developmental levels was pre-defined as the University wide scale for skills education that discerns attainment levels 1, 2 and 3. Next to these levels the rubric enables to add additional written feedback for each criterion. See Fig. 2.6.

**Performance Descriptors (*Rubric Cells*)** The '*micro-skills*' as criteria were operationalized to observable behaviours that students—based on experience of the teachers in the project team and already existing material in the university—tend to display while collaborating in courses of their BSc program. Adequate behaviours were used as descriptions of the middle level that students need to meet. Aspects that students tend to struggle with were used to explicate the lowest level and excellent behaviours were used to describe the highest level. This way the three different levels of development of student performances were defined.

**Construction and Fine-Tuning with Other Teachers** The resulting rubric was firstly used to discuss with teachers how collaboration is addressed in their course: what micro-skills? What levels? This helped to design learning activities that could be integrated within particular courses and talk about alignment between different courses resulting in an intended longitudinal learning trajectory extending over 2 or 3 years. During this whole first round of trying out, feedback on the rubric, its micro-skills and level descriptions was collected. This led to some small changes in the collaboration rubric for the next academic year. Descriptions were adapted to make them more distinctive (both between rows (criteria) and columns (levels)) and to minimize the overlap and redundancy that was experienced initially.

**Communication to Students** As explained, the learning activities to practice collaboration skills are embedded in different courses in the programs and as such interrelated to the course content. The information on these learning activities and the rubric are presented to students in the online learning environment (Brightspace). The rubric is also available as a Word document that students can use for self-assessment and reflection.

## 2.3.3 Use of the Rubric in Practice

Evaluation of collaboration skills is not based on a single assignment. In this skills learning trajectory, the rubric is constantly used as the underlayer to evaluate students' performance and growth, give feedback and set new goals. Students, peers, teachers and student assistants all use the same rubric throughout the program. It focuses on development and depends on multiple direct observations and skills-related assignments integrated in several courses of the program. During this skill development trajectory, students gather these experiences and proofs in a portfolio (in Brightspace) and reflect periodically on progression in their personal development on communication skills to set and adapt personal learning goals.

**Grading and Feedback** Whether students reached the required level of collaboration skills is evaluated and graded as pass or fail at the end of the learning trajectory. The student uses the feedback gathered throughout the skills development trajectory in a personal reflection assignment. So rubric scores as such are not used for grading collaboration skills but are used as information to underpin the students conclusion on his own development. Plan for the future is to add a final group assignment where students are observed in a challenging collaborative assignment that is video recorded and graded. As additional feedback to the level score, the last column of the rubric is used to write an explanation that underpins this score. During practice and training of collaboration skills, feedback is provided with the rubric as a guidance. In addition, trained student assistants annually provide feedback to students self-assessment and to the reflection on their progression in the development of collaboration skills and the personal learning goals they formulated. This feedback is provided as remarks in the documents uploaded in Brightspace. In addition, student assistants give feedback on the written feedback that students provide to peers.

**Evaluation and Improvement** For evaluation of collaboration skills multiple voices are an asset rather than a complication. So for feedback by peers in group work some variation between individuals feedback is considered as rich information instead of 'noise' that should be avoided. The student assistants, who do most of the more formal assessment, are trained by educational experts in collaboration skills and giving feedback. Practicing with the rubric is part of these training meetings.

## 2.4 Rubric for Clinical Skills

| Rubric | Rubric for clinical skills |
|---|---|
| Educational program | Bachelor Medicine |
| Faculty | Radboud University Medical Center |
| University | Radboud University, Nijmegen, The Netherlands |
| Course? | Practice and Principles of Medicine |
| Course coordinator | E. Rasenberg, MSc (general practitioner and coordinator skills and communication education Radboudumc), and L. Rietveld, MSc (general practitioner and teacher Radboudumc) |
| Written by | Dr. H. Pluk (teacher and curriculum coordinator Radboudumc) |

## Self-Assessment form for collaboration skills

Student name.................................................................... Date....................

*Mark (by underlining, circling, ticking) for each microskill which level you find applicable for yourself when you look back at previous experiences with group experiences of BVG year-1 and briefly explain why you chose this level. In addition, see whether you can already identify your qualities and challenges (focus points) for future collaborations. Formulate 2 SMART personal learning goals from these focus points (for instruction and more information open the folder Supportive skills - Reflection) that you are motivated for to work on during this academic year. Note them down underneath the table.*

Performance levels for collaboration skills
After successful completion of this year students are expected to be able to....

| | Level | Level-1 | Level-2 | Level-3 | Explanation |
|---|---|---|---|---|---|
| | Microskill | Basic group work, having meetings and contributing to group assignment. | Group work in courses. | Group work in multidisciplinary teams. | |
| C1 | Structuring meetings and group work (setting objectives) | Know how to structure meetings and group work when assigned a group assignment | Structure meetings and group work and set objectives guided by the teacher | Structure meetings and group work and set objectives on their own | |
| C2 | Executing team role and corresponding tasks (chair, secretary, member) | Know what the team roles and corresponding tasks are about and understand the value of each role | Execute at least one of the group roles and corresponding tasks supported by the group members | Execute all group roles and corresponding tasks supported by the group members | |
| C3 | Giving and receiving feedback | Understand the guidelines for giving and receiving feedback | Apply the guidelines for giving and receiving feedback | Proactively ask for feedback and use it for personal improvement, as well as give feedback constructively | |

## 2.4 Rubric for Clinical Skills

| | | | | |
|---|---|---|---|---|
| C4 | Contributing to the discussion content-wise | Select input from different sources and share this information with the group | Select input from different sources and share the relevant information with the group | Select input from different sources and share the relevant information with the group. Structure this information to integrate all relevant input |
| C5 | Contributing to the discussion process-wise (listening; speaking; argumenting) | Listen (pro-)actively and ask clarifying questions when needed. Speak up and give arguments for own input | Listen (pro-)actively and ask clarifying questions when needed. Speak up and give arguments for own input. Discuss constructively when different opinions arise | Listen (pro-)actively and ask clarifying questions when needed. Speak up and give arguments for own input. Discuss constructively when different opinions arise. Involve all group members in the discussion |
| C6 | Group processes and dealing with them (dealing with diversity; conflict handling; decision-making; responding to group dynamics) | Recognize the group dynamics and recognize their own role in that | Explain the group dynamics and acknowledge their own role in that. Stay engaged during all peaks and troughs, with the intention to continuously contribute to the group process in an effective way | Analyse the group dynamics and consciously choose their own role in that. Address diversity, conflict or decision-making, with the intention to resolve it |
| C7 | Being open to multiple perspectives and showing a learning attitude | Show an open attitude towards different perspectives of group members | Show an open attitude towards different perspectives of group members and listen actively to understand these perspectives | Show an open attitude towards different perspectives of group members and listen actively to learn from these perspectives. Ask proactively to get an overview of all perspectives |

**Fig. 2.6** Criteria and performance levels for collaboration skills, illustrating the developmental path. (Courtesy of Suzet Zijlstra, MSc, MA, Dr. Judith Gulikers and Dr.ir.ing. Carla Oonk (Education and Learning Sciences), in collaboration with Dr. Wilma Steegenga (Nutrition and Health), Dr. Marjolijn Coppens (Biology) and Inge Palm (Animal Sciences), Wageningen University and Research, The Netherlands)

**2 Personal SMART learning goals for academic year-2:**

1. ..................................................................................................................

2. ..................................................................................................................

**Fig. 2.6** (continued)

## 2.4 Rubric for Clinical Skills

### 2.4.1 Context in Which the Rubric Is Developed and Used

The curriculum of the bachelor's program Medicine at Radboud University Medical Centre (Radboudumc) has been completely revised in 2015. In this revision learning trajectories have been created that stimulate the longitudinal development of students in theoretical mechanisms of health and disease, scientific reasoning, professional and personal development and clinical skills. In the clinical skills learning trajectory *'Practice and Principles of Medicine'* the main learning objective is *'to develop general skills required to provide personalized care and to obtain insight in the relevant backgrounds'*. In this learning trajectory clinical skills like physical examination techniques (psychomotor skills; e.g. abdominal or thorax examination, inspection of head and neck, blood pressure measurement) are demonstrated, practiced and assessed. Also the skills for communication and consultation to determine a clinical diagnosis are learned by practicing with peers and simulated patients (people trained to portray real patients with a clinical problem). Assessment in this learning trajectory, with over 300 students each year, is performed via demonstration of the required skills in practice tests (standardized patient examinations) with simulators and simulated patients. A large number of clinicians are involved in the education and assessment. In order to reach a more uniform and objective assessment, rubrics were developed. These enable students to get insight in the skill levels required, obtain feedback and guide the many involved clinicians in assessment. In Fig. 2.7 an example is given of one of the psychomotor skills rubrics (for thorax examination) and in Fig. 2.8 the communication and consultation rubric that is used for assessment at the end of the bachelor's program is depicted.

### 2.4.2 Construction of the Rubric to Assess Clinical Skills

#### 2.4.2.1 Rubric for Psychomotor Skills

**Setting Criteria (*Rubric Rows*)** Rubric criteria, such as for example inspection of the thorax or use of percussion techniques in an examination of the posterior thorax (see Fig. 2.7), were set based upon detailed clinical protocols that were developed in the revision of the curriculum. For each particular physical examination or psychomotor skill to be learned, detailed protocols were written (based upon textbook protocols or current clinical practice at Radboudumc) in order to teach these skills to all students in a uniform way by all the teachers involved.

**Rating Scale (*Rubric Columns*)** For all rubrics in the clinical skills learning trajectory the rating scales *'insufficient'*, *'sufficient'* and *'good'* were chosen. Since it appeared already quite a challenge to describe each of these scales, further fine-tuning was not deemed appropriate. For feedback purposes a more fine-grained scale is also not of great value for further learning.

| Thorax examination rubric (level end of year 1 BSc Medicine (Q4)) | | | |
|---|---|---|---|
| **Criterion** | **Insufficient** | **Sufficient** | **Good** |
| Introduces him/her | Not executed | Lacks one or more items OR not polite | Name and function (medicine student); makes proper contact |
| Hand disinfection | Not executed | Lacks one or more steps | Uses alcohol twice (upon entering room and after examination); alcohol is evaporated before examination starts |
| Inspection thorax posterior | Not executed | Lacks one or more items OR one or more items not executed properly | Describes inspection; stands directly behind patient; patient is standing or sitting on examination table. Addresses: skin abnormalities, presence of dyspnoea, thorax shape, respiration (frequency, symmetry, muscle use, sound) |
| Percussion thorax posterior | Not executed | Lacks one or more steps OR one or more steps not executed properly | Systematic percussion: alternating left/right; top to bottom and flanks. Afterwards borders of lungs (both sides) and displacement properties |
| Percussion technique | Not executed or erroneous technique | Partly not executed OR erroneous technique | Flat hand, fingers parallel to ribs, audible percussion. Determines borders of lungs and displacement properties |
| Auscultation | Lacks multiple steps or not executed properly | Lacks one or few steps or not executed properly | Systematic auscultation: alternating left/right; top to bottom and flanks; minimal 8 spots per lung (including flanks); minimum one complete breath per spot |
| Instruction patient to sigh | No instruction | Lacks a step | Gets patient to sigh with opened mouth |
| Answering of questions | No correct questions or due to time limits no questions asked | One question correct | All questions correct |
| General impression | Insufficient | Sufficient | Good |
| Score | Insufficient | Sufficient | Good |

**Fig. 2.7** Example rubric psychomotor skills (thorax posterior examination; year 1 BSc Medicine; 2020). (Courtesy of L. Rietveld, MSc (translated from Dutch))

## 2.4 Rubric for Clinical Skills

|  | **Insufficient** | **Sufficient** | **Good** |
|---|---|---|---|
| **Reason for patient visit** | The question of the patient is not clear | The question of the patient is partly clear | The question of the patient is clear |
| **Biopsychosocial context of patient** | The context of the patient is not sufficiently discussed. Not all elements of the SCEBS method are discussed AND the obtained information is too superficial leading to a lack of relevant information | The context of the patient is sufficiently discussed. BUT not all elements of the SCEBS method are discussed OR the obtained information is superficial leading to a lack of relevant information | The context of the patient is well discussed. All elements of the SCEBS method are discussed AND the obtained information is informative, relevant and complete |
| **Investigation of complaint/problem** | Does not select relevant complaints/problems to investigate further | Does select relevant complaints/problems to investigate further BUT does not go in sufficient detail | Does select relevant complaints/problems to investigate further AND goes into sufficient detail |
| **Medical content** | Does not ask for proper symptom(s) OR misses more than 2 items in correct symptom | Does ask for proper symptom(s) BUT misses 2 items | Does ask for proper symptom(s), is complete OR misses only 1 item |
| **Logical reasoning** | Follows mainly checklists and does not show logical thinking | Follows many checklists but also shows logical thinking and follow-up questions. The conversation is not yet fluent | Shows logical thinking and follow-up questions. Questioning leads to a logical and fluent conversation |
| **Addresses patient signals** | Does not name signals patient is giving | Does only sometimes name signals patient is giving OR names signals in an uncomfortable way for the patient | Does name signals patient is giving in a comfortable way |
| **Shows empathy** | Does not or only minimal show empathy for the patient | Does show empathy for the patient BUT clumsy or not at appropriate time | Does show empathy for the patient in a comfortable way |
| **Patient involvement** | No collaboration between physician and patient | Some collaboration between physician and patient BUT the physician should give more room for questions/ideas of the patient AND/OR should take the patient more along in his/her reasoning | Good collaboration between physician and patient. Physician gives room for questions/ideas of the patient and reasons out loud and explains his/her reasoning |
| **Structure: summaries; markings; logical order; timing** | The mentioned skills are not used sufficiently leading to a non-structured conversation | The mentioned skills are used BUT the conversation is not clearly structured all the time | Using the mentioned skills a structured conversation is held with the patient |
| **Grade** | | | |
| **Feedback** | | | |

**Fig. 2.8** Rubric communication and consultation (Anamnesis, year 3 BSc Medicine; 2020). (Courtesy of E. Rasenberg, MSc. (translated from Dutch))

**Performance Descriptors (*Rubric Cells*)** The performance description approach for each cell was uniform for all developed psychomotor skills rubrics. Correct and complete execution of the basic steps from the detailed clinical protocol of a particular psychomotor skill was set as '*good*'. For the cells in the scales '*sufficient*' and '*insufficient*', an incomplete or technically incorrect execution was in place.

**Construction and Fine-Tuning with Other Teachers** The protocols of all to be learned psychomotor skills, such as abdominal examination, inspection of the head and neck, blood pressure measurement, and assessment of heart and lung sound, of the Bachelor Medicine were written down by a small dedicated team of clinical teachers, based upon physical examination textbooks and protocols in use at Radboudumc. Based upon these protocols all rubrics (15 in total) were developed by the same team. Since many teachers are involved in the actual assessment of the psychomotor skills, and not all have a similar experience in teaching or assessment, *'knowledge clips'* were produced to instruct all teachers about the use of these rubrics and the clinical protocols involved. Teachers need to watch these before instruction and assessment. In addition, in yearly teacher meetings a rubric is filled in together and discussed. In case of protest of students on a particular assessment, these comments are discussed with the involved teachers which also leads to fine-tuning of scoring. The involved teachers of the psychomotor skills grow as a team in the use of these rubrics. Special attention is, however, needed for new teachers.

**Communication to Students** Psychomotor skills rubrics are presented to students only in the first part of their bachelor's program (until the third semester). Students practice physical examinations using these rubrics and feedback is given. In a lecture the use of the rubrics and its feedback purpose is explained to students. In the second part of their bachelor's program, only detailed clinical protocols for each physical examination are given to students, in order to train students to use these kinds of protocols. Assessors are provided with all rubrics in all bachelor phases for scoring and feedback purposes of the psychomotor skills.

### 2.4.2.2 Rubric for Communication and Consultation Skills

Next to psychomotor skills also communication and consultation skills are assessed during standardized patient examinations in the clinical skills learning trajectory. The criteria and performance descriptors for rubrics assessing these skills, such as showing empathy and logical reasoning (see Fig. 2.8), were set by a small group of dedicated experienced teachers. Based upon their experiences in clinical education, inspired by similar rubrics available in literature, on-line or gathered via colleagues at other institutions these rubrics were developed, used and adapted during use in the first years of the new curriculum. The communication and consultation rubric is the same in year 2 and 3 and very identical in year 1 of the Medical bachelor's degree program (the rubric of year 1 is focused strongly on the technical aspects of asking questions during a consult). The level of the skills assessment is altered by increasing the difficulty and/or complexity of the simulated, standardized patient examination in later years. For example, a simple rhinitis is assessed in the first year while a complex pulmonary inflammation may be assessed in the third year.

In the first months of their bachelor, students are asked to set and discuss the criteria and rating scale for a rubric concerning the skill *'showing empathy'*. In this way the setting of rubrics and its use for feedback purposes is highlighted in the clinical skills learning trajectory. All rubrics for assessment of communication and consultation skills are made known to students at the beginning of each academic year. All teachers involved in assessment are also involved in teaching of communication and consultation skills. A practice standardized patient examination is assessed and discussed together. This meeting is used to fine-tune scoring and gather feedback for adaptations and improvements of the rubric by the coordinating teacher each year.

### 2.4.3 Use of the Rubrics in Practice

Since both psychomotor skills and communication and consultation rubrics are used for assessment in live standardized patient examinations (that last about 9 min) for many students (over 300 each time) the scoring of these rubrics needs to be fast and easy. Scoring and giving feedback needs to be done directly and in a very short amount of time after and during skills demonstration. Digital assessment with these rubrics using iPads and the program LimeSurvey (Limesurvey.org), taking care of not too complicated rubrics with short text items in all cells, is needed in order to achieve this.

**Grading and Feedback** Just counting all rubric criteria was sometimes in contradiction with the overall expert judgement of assessors about the level a student reached in his/her demonstration of clinical skills. Even if criteria are set very carefully, addressing most important elements, not all behaviour during a standardized patient examination can be captured in a rubric. This was experienced in use of both the psychomotor skills and communication and consultation rubrics. Also differences were noted in the individual assessment of criteria by different assessors while the overall assessment of a student was scored with a similar final grade. Although measures to enhance uniformity are in place (as described above), some variation in what assessors observe and value is inevitable and part of professional practice as well; it is viewed as relevant information rather than 'noise' (van der Vleuten et al., 2010). These experiences lead to the choice that the final grade of each assessment is not directly mathematically calculated by scoring of the cells in the rubric. The assessors give a final grade or score insufficient/sufficient/good, taking into account the rubric scores and their professional experience.

For giving of narrative feedback an extra box was included in the communication and consultation rubric. In general, giving and receiving feedback is a very important item in the clinical skills learning trajectory. After each standardized patient examination with simulated patients, feedback is given by peers (e.g. by using the digital video program TrainTool (n.d.)) and self-reflection is stimulated. In an intensive collaboration with the learning trajectory 'Professional and personal development' peer feedback and self-reflection is further developed and practiced.

**Evaluation and Improvement** In general teachers are content with the use of the clinical skills rubrics. Especially, in the psychomotor skills assessments with many students and many teachers it is of help to obtain a more balanced grading and to give feedback to students in a fast and efficient way. The relation between the assessment of the rubric cells and the final grade is an issue the coordinating teacher would still like to improve.

Teachers noticed that the psychomotor skills rubrics strongly direct the learning attitude of students and many times students only used the rubric as a checklist. In order to reflect the clinical work setting better and to stimulate students to critically address clinical protocols themselves, they have chosen to provide students only with the clinical protocols in later bachelor periods. The actual rubric for assessment is then only provided to teachers.

In the first years of using the communication and consultation rubric, teachers noticed that students tended to use the provided rubric to 'tick-off, one-by-one' all listed criteria which sometimes led to a very artificial conversation with a (simulated) patient. By adding and using more narrative feedback this undesired behaviour is addressed and discussed with students. This narrative feedback is now seen as the most important aspect in the use of these rubrics, to give feedback about the more 'soft' communication skills such as word phrasing and non-articulate behaviour.

## References

Brightspace, D2L Corporation. (n.d.). https://www.d2l.com/
Campbell, N., Gaston, A., Gray, C., Rush, E., Maddison, R., & Prapavessis, H. (2016). The Short Questionnaire to Assess Health-Enhancing (SQUASH) physical activity in adolescents: A validation using doubly labeled water. *Journal of Physical Activity and Health, 13*(2), 154–158.
de Vegt, F., Otten, J. D. M., de Bruijn, D. R. H., Pluk, H., van Rooij, I. A. L. M., & Oostendorp, T. F. (2021). Research in action—Students' perspectives on the integration of research activities in undergraduate biomedical curricula. *Medical Science Educator, 31*, 371–374. https://doi.org/10.1007/s40670-021-01228-8
Eriksson, N., Macpherson, J. M., Tung, J. Y., Hon, L. S., Naughton, B., Saxonov, S., Avey, L., Wojcicki, A., Pe'er, I., & Mountain, J. (2010). Web-based, participant-driven studies yield novel genetic associations for common traits. *PLoS Genet, 6*(6), e1000993.
TrainTool. (n.d.). https://www.faculty.nl/en/traintool-app/
Turn-it-in. (n.d.). https://www.turnitin.com/
van der Vleuten, C. P. M., Schuwirth, L. W. T., Scheele, F., Driessen, E. W., & Hodges, B. (2010). The assessment of professional competence: Building blocks for theory development. *Best Practice & Research Clinical Obstetrics & Gynaecology, 24*, 703–719. https://doi.org/10.1016/j.bpobgyn.2010.04.001
Wendel-Vos, G. C., Schuit, A. J., Saris, W. H., & Kromhout, D. (2003). Reproducibility and relative validity of the short questionnaire to assess health-enhancing physical activity. *Journal of Clinical Epidemiology, 56*(12), 1163–1169.

# Chapter 3
# Perspectives on Rubrics

## Contents

| | | |
|---|---|---|
| 3.1 | Perspectives of Students.................................................................... | 41 |
| 3.2 | Perspectives of Educational Advisors..................................................... | 43 |
| 3.3 | Perspectives of Teachers..................................................................... | 44 |
| 3.4 | Perspectives of Curriculum Coordinators and Managers............................... | 46 |
| References............................................................................................ | | 48 |

**Abstract** Here we describe the perspectives of the different stakeholders in using rubrics for assessment and feedback. First and foremost, the perspectives of students as the group that directly benefits from the feed-up, feedback and feed-forward properties of rubrics are highlighted. After a perspective on the supporting role of educational advisors, considerations for teachers are listed. Do's and don'ts in the grading and feedback aspects of rubrics are described as support and practical tips for teachers wanting to implement rubrics in their education. Last, perspectives of curriculum managers are included, since also these stakeholders have their own role in stimulating good use of rubrics, for example by facilitating the long-term use of rubrics and by underlining the formal role of the examination board in warranting assessment quality in programs and courses.

## 3.1 Perspectives of Students

When talking about the implementation of rubrics, focus often is on the teachers and assessors. However, it is the students that should be central in a discussion on rubrics (or, for that matter, any educational measure). As already mentioned in Chap. 1, using rubrics clearly can have many benefits for students, as feed-up, feedback and feed-forward, facilitating self-assessment and peer review and enhancing transparency and consistency of assessment procedures. But these benefits are not intrinsic qualities of a rubric per se, and neither is a rubric in all circumstances the best tool to achieve these (see also perspectives of teachers for the latter). We will walk you through these different aspects to indicate some important pitfalls and considerations from the students' point of view.

**Personal Quote Student**

> Rubrics provide me with a good overview of the structure I need to use when writing a report. I often score my own work with the rubric to get an idea of how well I performed and to see where improvements can be made.

**Feed-up** Because a rubric through the descriptors articulates how the assignment's product may look like, it can help students to envisage the product and understand what they are expected to deliver. Yet, in many cases the assignment will ask **students** to do something that is new to them, something they need to learn also through the assignment. A rubric alone may not be enough for students to recognize and understand this thing that is new to them. They will need guidance and support to become familiar with the concepts and context; otherwise the descriptions a rubric provide will not be understood and thus cannot serve as feed-up. Instead of starting with presenting a fixed rubric to students, starting with discussing together what characterizes a good quality product could be more engaging and also help to reveal misconceptions or relevant personal convictions. A rubric will bring the most benefit when it is an integral part of teaching and learning activities instead of just an 'add-on' to the assessment.

**Self-Assessment and Peer Feedback** As with feed-up, understanding what the rubric is about is required before students can use it to properly evaluate themselves or their peers. This doesn't mean only experts can use the rubric. The value of using the rubric for self-assessment and peer assessment is not only to get an impression of the quality of one's product. The use in itself is a way of getting to grips with the subject and thus part of the learning process (Filius, 2019). This may not be self-evident to students (and teachers); it may need some explaining and practice to entice students to use it as such.

**Feedback and Feed-Forward** By indicating what descriptors apply for a product, using a rubric is a very efficient means for assessors to provide feedback. The usefulness of this feedback for the student ofcourse depends largely on the clarity of the rubric. In many cases some additional personalized feedback that links info from the rubric to particularities of their specific product may greatly increase the usefulness for the student. And a rubric with pages of listing different criteria and a very fine-grained scale will likely be unmanageable and result in a cognitive overload that frustrates learning rather than helping it. Furthermore it is, as always, important that students have an opportunity to use the feedback to improve. And although there may be many such opportunities in a study program, they may not always be recognized as such by students (and teachers) if they see every assignment as a separate task to pass. Students may need help to understand the connections within a program in order to use input as feed-forward for further learning. If students are stimulated and guided to use feedback to define their personal strengths and weaknesses, they can define their own learning goals and take responsibility to develop on these throughout the program.

**Transparency** Using a rubric will not make assessment fully objective; some discussion on the interpretation of a rubric may remain both between students and teachers and amongst different assessors. There may often be more than one valid way of seeing things and increasingly so for assignments focusing on more complex tasks, related to real-life problems and contexts. Ruthlessly striving for objectivity to improve reliability of assessment may do much harm to the validity of the assessment (Schuwirth & van der Vleuten, 2012). Focusing on what is easily (quantitatively) objectified may obscure what is relevant to (qualitatively) measure for valid assessment.

**Personal Quotes from Students**

> Sometimes, I miss additional feedback after the rubric has been scored by the grader. Rubrics are useful for me as a student, provided that there is enough and clear information on what is expected from me.

> Rubrics provide me with a good overview of the structure I need to use when writing a report. I often score my own work with the rubric to get an idea of how well I performed and to see where improvements can be made.

## 3.2 Perspectives of Educational Advisors

Educational advisors are often asked by teachers to deliver examples of rubrics, or even to make a rubric. However tempting to delegate the time-consuming task of constructing a rubric to someone with didactical expertise in that matter, we would advise not to do so as a teacher. The way to go would probably be that the teacher or course coordinator keeps initiative throughout the construction, use and evaluation of the rubric. The role of the educational advisor would be to support this: sorting out expectations/objectives of the rubric, thus helping to make a blueprint, handing over examples, stimulating the teacher or course coordinator to seek co-creation with other teachers or students, giving feedback, stimulating integration of the rubric in the course, in existing learning trajectories and evaluation activities. As an educational advisor it seems tempting to push the swift use of rubrics in view of the many possibilities to foster learning mentioned in the manual such as facilitating feed-up, feedback and feed-forward, and self-assessment and peer assessment. Yet for a successful use of the rubric, it is important to temporize this process in order for the rubric to be supported and adopted by all the stakeholders involved.

**Personal Quotes from Educational Advisors**

> Don't make rubrics too complex, keep it simple.

> A deceptive claim for objective assessment?

> Difficult to make, convenient to use.

## 3.3 Perspectives of Teachers

**Using Rubrics for Assessment** Rubrics use with the purpose of scoring the students level, expressed in a grade, is still one of the major incentives for using rubrics. Yet in daily practice teachers sometimes experience rubrics' limitations, especially when grading. When using an (over)analytical or too detailed rubric, teachers find that the outcome (grade) doesn't always fit their own judgement. Many teachers therefore first grade using their own judgement and fill in the rubric accordingly, thus using the rubrics as backup. It does happen though that teachers base their scores only on their judgement and in doing so ignoring the rubric. This often happens when the use of a rubric has not been discussed or the rubric has been constructed by someone else than the teacher. In doing so the rubric has become useless for the purpose it was designed for in the first place. In such a context the rubric (or rubrics in general) becomes an instrument that is seen as playing a role in undermining the professional and intellectual competence of the teacher, a burden imposed by bureaucratic powers from above rather than being an asset for the teacher. In this situation it denies the teacher the possibility to grade more transparent, to better substantiate a given grade and facilitate feedback to students. First and foremost it might be wise to somewhat minimize the high expectations that are often linked to rubrics. Yes, it can be a good instrument to support teachers in grading students' performance, but no, do not see the rubric as a holy grail by using it as a recipe which automatically provides you with a reliable grade with one or more decimal places.

Given the fact that there are many practices where rubrics are experienced an asset in assessments, it seems that there are several dos and don'ts to consider in order for rubrics to deliver on its promise when assessing for a grade (see Table 3.1).

**Table 3.1** Some dos and don'ts using rubrics for grading

| | |
|---|---|
| **Construction** | Take a more holistic viewpoint in construction by adding an open text field to substantiate your grading and feedback instead of trying to catch all in the description of the cells, and/or adding complex mathematical schemes that result in a grade. |
| | Involve colleagues in constructing a rubric. Using a rubric designed by someone else often leads to neglect of the rubric to some degree. |
| **Usage** | Use the rubric for guidance purposes as well as for grading. |
| | Be aware that all assessors know the rubric by heart, especially when grading a presentation. This enables them to focus on observing the actual students' performance rather than reading the rubric and observing at the same time. |
| | Strive for more reliability through grading with more than one assessor. This will have a more positive effect on reliability instead of expecting reliability through objective assessment by using just the rubric itself. |
| **Evaluation** | Talk about grading with your colleagues and when doing so: look at the rubric, assignments and/or guiding process/activities at the same time. |
| | Test the rubric when it has been used by sampling, for instance, a few graded written products in the past. This could be a task done by a board of examiners or other teachers who are not directly involved in the products that were assessed with the rubric. Is the grade the same as the initially given grade or does it differ? And if so: what is the reason that the grade is different? This could give you important information to improve your rubric. |

## 3.3 Perspectives of Teachers

**Using Rubrics for Feedback** Feedback is considered to be a powerful stimulus for learners. The teacher plays an essential role in this. Does he or she really value the power of feedback? Students tend to notice quickly and accurately what the teacher considers important in reality. Furthermore when giving feedback the aspects of timing and the way feedback is delivered or triggered are important when using rubrics to enhance feedback for learning (Table 3.2).

### Personal Quotes from Teachers

> It is important to discuss the rubric and how it will be used with all assessors.
> Rubrics make the assessment of a paper less subjective.

> The use of a rubric gives students more direction to make an assignment properly and it helps you as a teacher to evaluate a student's assignment in a more standardized way.

> The use of rubrics greatly enhances the objectivity of my grades to students, however, it also reduces the flexibility in tweaking the grades when in doubt about a criterion.

> By providing the grading rubrics early to students and putting it into a practice assignment (prior to the grading product), students are forced to think critically about how to write and present results. This really gave rise to interesting questions and discussions on how to phrase certain concepts and how to report science in general.

**Table 3.2** Considerations related to rubrics for feedback

| | |
|---|---|
| Timing | When presenting the rubric to students before the start of a course, students might appreciate this because they seek for clues what exact behaviour or skill they need to show. When your goal with a rubric as a teacher is explicitly to enhance deeper learning though, this might not be the most effective strategy. This could lead to the following feedback of a teacher after a presentation: '...*thank you for your presentation of the case...so you did well, I could see that you read the rubric thoroughly in your preparation of your presentation.*' So handing over the rubric (shortly) before an assessment might lead to students learning (or copying) the rubric. This could be desirable, depending on your learning objectives. But if your learning objectives are more feedback driven, and exceed superficial learning, it is advised to plan the integration of the rubric more carefully and integrate the rubric in assignments throughout the course by means of using the rubric with self- and/or peer assessment, or even consider students co-creating your rubric. Feedback might just be more appreciated by students if they would not learn it by heart but would actually use the rubric actively. |
| The way feedback is delivered or triggered | Active usage by students and delivering feedback that truly supports students learning could also be done by rethinking the way feedback is delivered. You might want to ask students themselves on what aspect they want to receive feedback, or by whom they would prefer it from: the teachers and/or their peers. This not only activates their own thinking process but also solves the issue that a rubric in many cases never fully covers all individual feedback needs. So stop trying to cover all in the rubric but ask students themselves instead and use an open field in the rubric to give specific feedback to the student that cover subjects or aspects that are not described in the rubric but are important to one or more students. In doing so you also receive valuable information that you might want to add to the rubric. |

## 3.4 Perspectives of Curriculum Coordinators and Managers

In order to integrate and stimulate the use of rubrics in a curriculum, the management of an educational program needs to take a facilitating and stimulating role. As described in Chap. 1, rubrics serve different purposes for different stakeholders. For students a rubric helps to understand what they are expected to learn, it provides formative feedback and it informs how their product or performance is valued. Furthermore, self-assessment and peer evaluation are facilitated by the use of rubrics. For teachers rubrics provide guidance on how to evaluate and mark, resulting in a more transparent, valid and reliable assessment. All these aspects of the use of rubrics are of great value for curriculum coordinators/managers as the quality of learning may be enhanced.

Additionally, creating a rubric with a group of teachers will help in identifying the essentials of learning objectives and create a more uniform view among teachers of what needs to be taught and assessed in a course or curriculum. The (discussion about) longitudinal use of rubrics in a learning trajectory of the curriculum may thus strengthen the curriculum as a whole and not only benefit single courses. If rubrics are used in a longitudinal way, it is important to realize which criteria and which level is used to define the highest rating scales. Often these will be related to the learning objectives and expected end level of the curriculum. By varying in the weighing of criteria and scales or cut-off for grading, one can use a similar rubric in the beginning as well as end phase of a curriculum.

Aspects from a management perspective that need to be considered in order to introduce, stimulate and sustain the use of rubrics in an effective way are presented in Table 3.3. In conclusion, a joint effort of teachers and educational advisors steered by the curriculum management is required for success. In addition dialogue is needed with the examining board that has an independent role in safeguarding the quality of assessment. 'Early adaptors' of rubrics can serve as role models spreading the word to their peers about the benefits of using rubrics and how to go about its challenges. Giving sufficient time and support, sometimes combined with obligatory requests of an examination board, may be needed to let 'critical teachers' adopt rubrics.

## 3.4 Perspectives of Curriculum Coordinators and Managers

**Table 3.3** Considerations related to implementing rubrics in a curriculum

| | |
|---|---|
| **Introduction of the use of rubrics** | A way to stimulate and implement the use of rubrics and/or have rubrics in a learning trajectory built upon each other is by guiding the group of teachers in a specific course and/or learning trajectory to develop rubrics together, with advise of educational advisors. Revision of a curriculum can offer excellent opportunity to start with this on request of the curriculum management.<br>The management could ask a small group of teachers and educational advisors to develop a set of 'standard rubrics' for a number of regular assessments in a curriculum, for example an oral presentation or written report, and provide these rubrics as examples to teachers with the request to use these and offer help to personalize them for their own course if needed.<br>Creating an environment where teachers are stimulated to share educational best practices between each other will also help to build support for the use of rubrics. Showing practice examples and having teacher 'role models' may inspire colleagues who may be reluctant to adopt.<br>Introduction of rubrics can also be started via the instructions an examination board may give to examiners. By requesting the formulation of a rubric for summative assessments, the use of rubrics may become mandatory for specific assignments. Proper guidance of teachers in the construction and use of rubrics (by educational advisors and experienced peers) needs to be in place when this step is considered. |
| **Long-term use of rubrics** | In order to sustain an effective use of rubrics, and to prevent divergence of similar rubrics in a learning trajectory (if in place), regular evaluation of rubrics is required. Teacher meetings to calibrate the grading and feedback of rubrics in a particular course or learning trajectory should be stimulated/planned and may also be used to reflect on the longitudinal use.<br>After introduction of rubrics in a course or curriculum, long-term use is not automatically guaranteed. For example, new teachers or new assignments may be in place or first use of rubrics may be less positive than anticipated. Therefore, continuous stimulation, education of teachers and exchange of best practices about the use of rubrics need to be supported/organized by the management. In course and curriculum evaluations the use of rubrics should be a regular item to be evaluated with students and teachers. |
| **Feedback function** | Special attention needs to be given to how the feedback functions of rubrics can be integrated in the curriculum, see Sect. 1.2.5. For example, a timely introduction of rubrics to students, or the use of similar rubrics in a specific learning trajectory for similar assignments will enhance its feed-forward and feedback properties, respectively.<br>Exchange of ideas and discussion of teachers with educational advisers should be guided in order to raise awareness of these aspects by individual teachers. |
| **Support** | The digital educational platforms in use should be able to integrate the use of rubrics in an easy way. For example, in Brightspace rubrics can be fully integrated in assignments and scores are automatically kept. ICT support (such as a helpdesk and online instructions) to help teachers set up rubrics in these platforms is required and needs to be actively communicated to teachers. |
| **Educational culture** | If and how rubrics will be used to give feedback to students may be influenced by the educational culture. Assessment *for* learning (Martinez & Lipson, 1989) or assessment *of* learning may not be equally valued in all educational institutes worldwide. Also decisions about if and how to use a rubric for summative grading are influenced by the grading culture of the educational institute. For example: While in The Netherlands criterion-referenced assessment with an absolute cut-off (% of the maximum score of a rubric) is typically used, in the USA a norm-referenced approach where individual performance is compared with the performance of the group (% of the highest scoring students get a maximum grade) is common, resulting in different summative outcomes while using a similar rubric. |

# References

Filius, R. (2019). *Peer feedback to promote deep learning in online education; Unraveling the process*. PhD thesis. https://doi.org/10.13140/RG.2.2.28814.82247

Martinez, M. E., & Lipson, J. I. (1989). Assessment for learning. *Educational Leadership, 47*, 73–75.

Schuwirth, L. W. T., & van der Vleuten, C. P. M. (2012). Programmatic assessment and Kane's validity perspective. *Medical Education, 46*(1), 38–48.

# Conclusion

Years after their introduction, there is a large and still growing body of information on rubrics. Literature, literature reviews, theoretical frameworks that can be linked to rubrics, available practices and critical discussions can be found in abundance. Clearly rubrics play their part in the discourse of learning and assessment. This is no surprise because rubrics are appealing. Their appeal stems from rubrics being a concise one pager that offers much needed clarity when facing the challenges in the often complex reality of learning and assessment. At the same time, it is this attractiveness that can easily turn out to be fatal when considering the amount of dos and don'ts on different levels that need to be considered in order for rubrics to deliver on its promise. We will not give a recap of the amount of all relevant dos and don'ts here, but turn to the following question in this conclusion: what stands in our view out as the vital aspects that lead to enhanced learning and assessment through the use of rubrics?

## Rubrics Are a Team Effort

In all our practices and in literature the need for alignment is a key concept. In every phase this is the case: construction, use and evaluation. The 'not invented here' syndrome does seem to apply to rubrics. If seen as a mere one pager that can be easily passed on to another teacher, please reconsider your actions. Although teachers can teach the same content and learning goals, there is, to some extent, always a different dynamic within groups of students, and between the group and varying teachers. It turns out that rubrics are aiming at the heart of education: the delicate and important discourse among teachers and students. Therefore every teacher in the team needs to be involved. Co-creation and communication within a team of teachers to enhance learning and assessment is always important. This also holds for constructing, using, evaluating and improving rubrics: it is a team effort.

## Rubrics Take Time to Evolve

Considered as a time-consuming effort, especially in the construction phase, rubrics need constant maintenance because it proves to be difficult to get it right the first time. Moreover, considering the changes in student cohorts, teaching staff and organization, it is important to evaluate the rubric each year and adapt if needed to keep the instrument fit-for-purpose.

## Rubrics Require a Multi-perspective Approach and Commitment

To make the best out of using rubrics, it is worthwhile to invest time in contributions from different perspectives as described in this manual. Way to go would be to really overthink what the purpose is of using rubrics in your specific situation and taking time to think this through with students, teachers, educational advisors and management. The extra amount of time this takes will pay off, with rubrics being a helpful instrument for all stakeholders involved.

## Rubrics Need to Be Integrated in Education and Made Fit for Purpose

For rubrics to be effective you need to invest time to think through the way you integrate your rubric in your specific educational context. We have made some suggestions in this manual. Whatever choice you make in doing so, make it fit for purpose in your specific context. Optimizing assessment and enhancing learning are complex aims that are not always served with a quick fix. In our view this requires time and effort to make rubrics part of assessment and learning activities in a logical way.

We hope that this manual will help you to get started with rubric use or gives food for thought in further improving its current use in assessment and learning.

GPSR Compliance

The European Union's (EU) General Product Safety Regulation (GPSR) is a set of rules that requires consumer products to be safe and our obligations to ensure this.

If you have any concerns about our products, you can contact us on ProductSafety@springernature.com

In case Publisher is established outside the EU, the EU authorized representative is:

Springer Nature Customer Service Center GmbH
Europaplatz 3
69115 Heidelberg, Germany

**Batch number: 09151059**

Printed by Printforce, the Netherlands